Care for Pregnant Women who are Obese

Care for Pregnant Women who are Obese

edited by Yana Richens and Tina Lavender

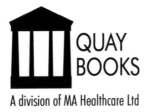

QUAY
BOOKS

A division of MA Healthcare Ltd

Note

Healthcare practice and knowledge are constantly changing and developing
as new research and treatments, changes in procedures, drugs and equipment become
available.

The author and publishers have, as far as is possible, taken care to confirm that the
information complies with

the latest standards of practice and legislation.

01269844.

Quay Books Division, MA Healthcare Ltd, St Jude's Church, Dulwich Road, London
SE24 0PB

British Library Cataloguing-in-Publication Data
A catalogue record is available for this book

© MA Healthcare Limited 2010
ISBN-10: 1 85642388 5; ISBN-13: 978 1 85642 388 3

Printed by CLE, Huntingdon, Cambridgeshire

1 4 SEP 2010

Contents

For Ruth who is good with words

Editors

Yana Richens RGN, RM, BSc (hons) MSc
Yana is a Consultant Midwife at University College London Hospital. She is a member of the Chief Nursing Officers national advisory group, providing specialist advice on black and ethnic minority issues in the NHS, and was the first midwife to be awarded the prestigious Mary Seacole Fellowship, an award made by the DoH. Yana was a member of the National Institute for Health and Clinical Excellence (NICE) guideline development group for the guideline on puerperal/perinatal mental health, and a member of the new NICE Guideline group for women with complex social problems. Yana is the Joint Editor-in-Chief of the *British Journal of Midwifery* and Associate Editor of the *African Journal of Midwifery*. In 2005 she co-founded the Female Genital Mutilation clinical guideline group. She leads a clinic for women with raised BMI at University College London Hospital and also has an interest in perineal trauma.

Tina Lavender PhD, MSc, RM
Tina Lavender is Professor of Midwifery at the University of Manchester. She also holds an honorary contract at St Mary's Hospital, Manchester. She leads a programme of research exploring maternal experiences, expectations and outcomes; her main research focus being the management of prolonged labour and partogram use. Tina has published extensively in this field. Tina's other area of expertise is maternity related public health; obesity is one of her areas of research activity. She is Joint Editor-in-Chief of the *British Journal of Midwifery*, Associate Editor of the *African Journal of Midwifery* and Associate Editor of the *Pregnancy and Childbirth* Group of the Cochrane Collaboration. Tina is an Honorary Fellow of the Royal College of Midwives and European Academy of Nurse Science.

List of Contributors

Rory M H Bell, MBBS, FRCA. Consultant Anaesthetist and Clinical Lead for Obstetric Anaesthesia University College London Hospitals NHS Foundation Trust.

Debra Bick RM, BA, MedSci, PhD. Professor of Evidence Based Midwifery Practice, King's College London.

Jason Cronje MBBS FRCA Anaesthetic SpR University College London Hospitals NHS Trust.

Laura de Rooy MBCHB, MRCP, FRCPCH Consultant Neonatologist and Care Group Lead, St George's Hospital, London.

Jane Hawdon MA, MBBS, MRCP, FRCPCH, PhD Consultant neonatologist and Director of Clinical Education, University College London Hospitals. Clinical lead, North Central London Perinatal Network.

Julie Hogg MSc, BSc (hons), Dip H.E, RM, RN, General Manager, Maternity & Neonatology, University College London Hospitals NHS Foundation Trust.

Alberic Fiennes BSc, MS, FRCS. Late Director of Baraitric Surgery, University College London Hosptitals NHS Trust, President British Obesity & Metabolic Surgery Society.

Christine Furber PhD, MSc, BSc, RN, RM, ADM, Cert Ed (FE), MTD Midwifery lecturer, School of Nursing Midwifery & Social Work The University of Manchester, Midwifery.

Cecilia Jevitt, CNM, PhD, ARNP, Associate Professor Midwifery and Nursing, University of South Florida Colleges of Nursing and Medicine, Tampa, Florida, USA.

Asma Khalil MB BCh, MD, MRCOG, Subspecialty Trainee in Maternal Fetal Medicine, Institute for Women's Health, University College London Hospitals.

Linda McGowan PhD, MSc, BSc, RN, RM, Lecturer in Women's Health, School of Nursing Midwifery & Social Work The University of Manchester, Midwifery.

Tracey A Mills BSc (Hons), RGN, RM, DPSM, MA, PhD Research Training Fellow, Maternal and Fetal Health Research Group, School of Clinical and Laboratory Sciences, The University of Manchester.

Pat O'Brien MB, BCh, BAO, FRCOG, FFSRH, FICOG, Consultant Obstetrician, Institute for Women's Health, University College London Hospitals.

Pranav Pandya BSc, MBBS, MRCOG, MD, Lead Consultant for Obstetrics & Fetal Medicine, University College London Hospitals NHS Foundation.

Daghni Rajasingam MA MRCOG, MBBS Consultant Obstetrician Guys and St Thomas' Hospital NHS Foundation Trust.

Hannah Rickard MBBS, BA(Oxon) Specialty Registrar in Obstetrics and Gynaecology Frimley Park Hospital NHS Foundation Trust.

Sheela Swamy MBBS, MRCOG, Senior Registrar, Department of Obstetrics and Gynaecology, Guys and St Thomas' Hospital.

Carina Venter B.Sc Dietetics, Post Grad Dipl in Allergy, PhD NIHR Post Doc Research Fellow, School of Health Sciences and Social Work, University of Portsmouth.

Foreword

The current obesity epidemic has lead to a substantial increase in the numbers of obese pregnant women. This means that obstetricians and midwives need to understand the effect of being obese on pregnancy and neonatal complications and outcomes. They also need to understand the implications of the obesity epidemic to service delivery. Obesity effects many elements of antenatal, intrapartum and postnatal care and is a multisystem disorder. This means that a multi-disciplinary approach is needed to manage the overweight and obese pregnant women appropriately. This book answers the challenge of collating the information needed to care for obese pregnant women. It is a clear, comprehensive, multi-disciplinary and well referenced exposition on obesity in pregnancy. Collecting this diverse information in one publication is timely and an invaluable resource for the practicing and academically active obstetricians, midwives and health service managers.

Siobhan Quenby

Professor of Obstetrics
University of Warwick

Chapter 1

Review of Obesity in Pregnancy in the UK

Tracey Mills

Introduction

There has been a well documented rise in the prevalence of obesity in the UK and current estimates suggest almost 25% of the adult population are obese. The consequences for public health are significant, including a rapidly rising incidence of type II diabetes. The cost to the NHS of treating the consequences of obesity has been estimated at £3.3-£3.7 billon per year, predicted to rise to £5 billion by 2025 (Foresight 2007). The cause(s) of the current epidemic of obesity are complex but are thought to relate to changes in energy intake and expenditure, notably physical activity. The negative impacts of obesity on the reproductive health of women are less well recognised. Obesity among pregnant women is becoming significantly more common and this is important to monitor because maternal obesity confers increased risks of poor pregnancy outcomes for both mother and baby.

The rising prevalence of obesity in the UK

Definition and classification of obesity

Obesity can be defined as an abnormal or excessive fat accumulation which presents a risk to health. Specifically, obesity is a major risk factor for numerous diseases including type II diabetes, coronary heart disease, hypertension, cancer and stroke (Must et al 1999). Currently, the recommended measure of obesity is body mass index (BMI), which is calculated as weight (in kilograms) divided by the square of the height (in metres). The classifications from the World Health Organisation (WHO 1997) for BMI are:
- BMI of 18.5-24.9 is healthy weight

- BMI of 25-29.9 is overweight
- BMI ≥ 30 is obese.

Obesity is sometimes further classified as:

- Class I (BMI 30-34.9)
- Class II (BMI 35-39.9)
- Class III (BMI ≥ 40; commonly termed 'morbid' obesity).

Body mass index is easy to calculate and is the recommended measure of obesity for use in early pregnancy (NICE 2008); however it has certain important limitations. Body mass index is not a direct measure of adiposity therefore individuals with a high lean muscle mass, such as athletes, may have a high BMI but low body fat. In most individuals BMI closely relates to total body fat, but it does not reflect differences in body fat distribution. Individuals with central (or abdominal) obesity, which is characterised by increased abdominal fat and waist size, are at greater risk of cardiovascular and metabolic diseases (Klein et al 2007).

Clinical studies have shown that waist circumference (WC) and waist to hip ratio (WHR) correlate closely with abdominal fat mass and may better predict obesity related disease risk than BMI (Yusuf et al 2005; Shen et al 2006). Waist Circumference and WHR, measured in early pregnancy, could be a useful tool for assessing the risk of obesity related complications. However, since both of these measures might be affected by fat accumulation in the first trimester, a thorough evaluation in pregnancy would be necessary to confirm whether they have advantages over BMI.

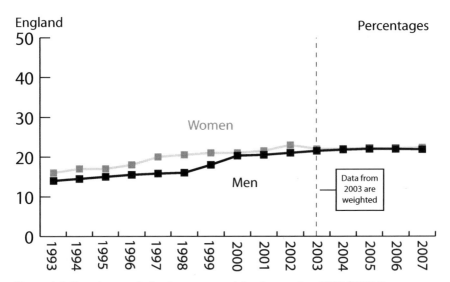

Figure 1.1 Prevalence of obesity among adults, by gender, 1993-2007. Source: Health Survey for England 2007- Latest Trends. Reproduced with permission from The NHS Information Centre.

Prevalence of obesity in the UK

The Health Survey for England (HSE), an annual survey of a representative sample of households in England, has reported a progressive increase in the proportion of adults who are obese (*Figure 1.1*). The prevalence of obesity has tripled from 8% in 1980 to 24% in 2007. In 2007, 65% of men and 56% of women were classified as overweight or obese. A corresponding decline has been observed in the proportion of the population with BMI in the normal range between 1993-2007, from 41% to 34% of men and from 50% to 42% of women (The NHS Information Centre 2009).

Additional analysis of the HSE reports a rise in obesity in the general population and has revealed variations according to age, ethnicity and social group. The prevalence of obesity increases with age in both men and women, and is lowest among 16-24 year olds. Of particular concern is the rapidly rising prevalence of overweight and obese children and adolescents. Obesity in children is also assessed using BMI, which is calculated in the same way as for adults. Rather than using set thresholds, comparison is made with typical values for other children of the same sex and age. BMI values are compared to percentiles; a BMI above the 95th percentile for sex and age is considered obese.. The HSE shows obesity in 2-15 year olds increased from 11% to 17% of boys and 12% to 16% of girls from 1995 to 2007 (*Figure 1.2*). Prevalence is higher in older children; 25% of 11-15 year olds were reported to be obese in 2004 (The NHS Information Centre 2009). Furthermore, obesity in adolescence tends to persist into adult life; the risk being greater

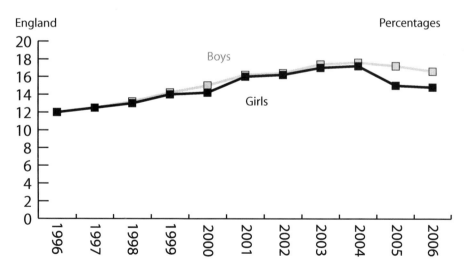

Figure 1.2 Obesity prevalence among children aged 2-15, 1995-2007. Source: Health Survey for England 2007- Latest Trends. Reproduced with permission The NHS Information Centre.

if at least one parent is obese (Guo et al 2002). A recent longitudinal study of 5863 UK school children from the age of 11-12 demonstrated that children who are obese after the age of 11 are significantly more likely to be obese as adults (Wardle et al 2006).

The HSE data also suggests that the incidence of obesity varies by ethnic group. In 2004, obesity among black Caribbean and Irish men was similar to the general population, while Pakistani, Indian, Bangladeshi and Chinese men had a lower prevalence. However, in black Caribbean, black African and Pakistani women the prevalence was higher than in the general population (*Table 1.1*).

The threshold categories recommended for BMI were developed for white Caucasian populations and there is increasing awareness that these may be inappropriate for other ethnic groups. For example, two studies (Forouhi and Sattar 2006; Mukhopadhyay et al 2006) have shown that South Asians have different body fat distribution to Caucasians. South Asians tend to have thinner limbs, but have higher waist to hip ratio and subscapular to triceps skinfold ratio than Caucasians, indicating greater central obesity. South Asians have also been shown to have a greater percentage of body fat than Caucasians. These differences in physical characteristics are thought to contribute to the higher rates and earlier onset of diabetes and cardiovascular disease in South Asians compared to Europeans. The WHO now recommends that South Asians be considered overweight at BMI ≥23.5 and obese at BMI ≥27.5 (WHO 2004).

The prevalence of raised waist circumference in men and women by equivalised household income (a measure of household income which takes account of the number of people living in each household) in 2007 is shown in *Figure 1.3*. There was no relationship between obesity and household incomes for men. In contrast however, women from the lowest income quintile had the

Table 1.1 % Adults by ethnicity and gender with BMI >30 compared with the general population. Data derived from Health Survey for England 2004: The health of ethnic minority groups. Reproduced with permission The NHS Information Centre.

	Men (N=4288)	Women (N=5322)
Black Caribbean	25%	32%
Black African	17%	38%
Pakistani	15%	28%
Indian	14%	20%
Bangladeshi	6%	17%
Chinese	6%	8%
Irish	25%	21%
General Population	23%	23%

highest prevalence of raised waist circumference, with the lowest prevalence in the highest income quintile (The NHS Information Centre 2009). Similarly, women in the lowest income quintile also had the highest mean BMI. The reasons why socio-economic deprivation increases obesity amongst women, but not men, is not understood but requires further study if effective strategies to reduce obesity in the future are to be developed.

Causes of obesity

On an individual level, obesity is the result of chronic energy imbalance which develops when energy intake exceeds energy expenditure. Unfortunately, relatively small excess intake or decreased energy expenditure can lead to substantial weight gain over a period of time. For example, an excess intake of 100 kcal/day (the equivalent of two plain biscuits) would lead to an extra 36 500 kcal/year which equates to over 5 kg of weight gain, mostly stored as fat. Over five years this would equate to a gain of approximately 25 kg. A woman who weighed 65 kg with a BMI of 23 would then weigh 90 kg with a BMI >30, classifying her as obese.

The factors which regulate adiposity and weight control are not fully understood. Studies of identical twins have demonstrated that significant differences in BMI are rare, suggesting that genetic background is important (Pietilainen et al 2004). However, purely genetic causes are rare. Single gene disorders, including mutations in the fat derived hormone leptin and its receptor, pro-opiomelanocortin (POMC) and the melanocortin 4 receptor (MC4R), produce extreme early onset obesity, but these disorders account for less than 5% of all severe obesity (O'Rahilly et al 2003). Defective genes are also responsible for syndromes such as Prader Willi and Bardet-Biedl,

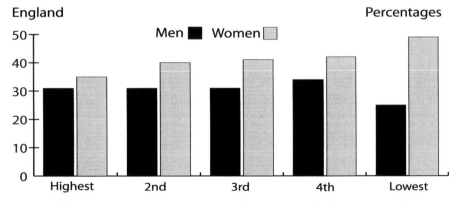

Figure 1.3 Prevalence of raised waist circumference by equivalised household income and gender, 2007. Source: Health Survey for England 2007. Reproduced with permission The NHS Information Centre.

which often feature obesity as part of their clinical presentation, but how these genetic abnormalities lead to obesity is not yet understood.

While genetic background is undoubtedly important in determining individual propensity to gain weight, it cannot explain the current obesity epidemic. Rather, the primary driver of the rise in obesity over the last two decades is thought to be changes in our lifestyles and surroundings which have altered food intake and decreased physical activity creating an 'obesogenic environment'.

Developed countries, including the UK, have witnessed changing patterns of energy intake such as a rise in food consumption outside the home and a growing availability and accessibility to calorie dense foods. Specifically, obesity has been linked to increased intake of sugary soft drinks (Malik et al 2006) and large portions of fast food intake (Pereira et al 2005).

There has also been a general decline in physical activity, with environmental changes favouring increased car use over walking and a trend towards sedentary leisure activities, such as television watching and computing. The HSE, consistent with other studies, has also reported that women are less likely to be physically active at all ages than men. In 2006, 50% of men aged 16-34 met the physical activity recommendations (undertaking at least 30 minutes of at least moderate intensity activity 5 days a week) while only 34% of women aged 16-34 met this target (The NHS Information Centre 2009).

Obesity in pregnancy

There is a lack of national statistics concerning the prevalence of obesity in pregnant women in the UK. The Confidential Enquiry into Maternal and Child Health (CEMACH) is currently conducting a major obesity project which will determine the prevalence of BMI >35 in pregnancy. The prevalence of obesity in women of reproductive age is rising according to the HSE which reported in 2003 that 17.8% of women aged 16-44 were obese (DH 2004). Several UK studies have described an increase in the numbers of women who are obese at the start of pregnancy. In Cardiff, between 1990-1999 the rate of obesity in primigravid women more than doubled from 3.2% to 8.9% (Usha Kiran et al 2005). The prevalence of women with BMI >30 in Glasgow increased from 9.4% in 1990 to 18.9% in 2002/4 (Kanagalingam et al 2005). A similar increase from 9.9% to 16% was reported in a retrospective study of 36 821 women in Middlesbrough from 1990-2004, which also reported a significant association between obesity and residence in an area of high social deprivation (Heslehurst et al 2007). A model based on the data collected for this study has predicted that 22% of pregnant women will be obese by 2010. Overall, these studies indicate that the trend towards increased rates of obesity in the general population is also present among pregnant women (Heslehurst et al 2007).

Consequences of Maternal Obesity in Pregnancy

The rapid increase in obesity among pregnant women in the last two decades is an important public health issue. Large epidemiological studies consistently report that obesity has significant negative impacts on the short and long term health of the mother and her baby. In the triennium 2000-2003 CEMACH reported that obesity was a factor in 35% of maternal deaths (Lewis, Drife 2004). The Perinatal Mortality Report 2005 found 30% of the women who had a stillbirth or neonatal death were obese (CEMACH 2007).

Prepregnancy obesity vs weight gain in pregnancy?

The complications associated with obesity generally relate to prepregnancy obesity, rather than excessive weight gain during pregnancy which results in a woman of healthy weight becoming obese (Catalano 2007). There are no current national guidelines for weight gain in pregnancy in the UK; recommendation are often based on the US Institute of Medicine (IOM) guidelines published in 1990 (Institute of Medicine, 1990). The IOM proposed a weight gain during pregnancy of:

- 11.5-16 kg for healthy weight women
- 7-11.5 kg for overweight women
- at least 7 kg for obese women.

However these guidelines were aimed at reducing the risk of fetal growth restriction rather than minimising obesity related complications and are currently under review.

It is not clear that obese women gain more weight in pregnancy than those of healthy prepregnancy weight. A small prospective US study reported no difference in the gain of fat mass or lean muscle mass during gestation between normal weight and obese women (Ehrenberg et al 2003). However, the increase in the percentage of body fat was greater in normal weight women. Interestingly, this study demonstrated differences in the distribution of fat mass between normal weight and obese women. There was a general increase in subcutaneous fat in the central region (between the mid thorax and upper thigh), but normal weight women gained more peripheral (biceps and triceps) subcutaneous fat than obese women.

Little is known about changes in abdominal fat during pregnancy.

Longitudinal ultrasound assessment in women of healthy BMI demonstrated evidence for a greater increase in abdominal fat compared to subcutaneous fat over gestation (Kinoshita and Itoh 2006). Abdominal fat accrual has not been investigated in overweight and obese women during pregnancy but could be an important determinant of the risk of complications as increased abdominal fat in non pregnant individuals is strongly associated with poor health outcomes.

Maternal antenatal risks

Miscarriage

Obese women are at increased risk of poor pregnancy outcomes from early gestation. Obese women who conceive naturally are at increased risk of early miscarriage (odds ratio [OR] 1.2, 95% confidence interval [CI] 1.01-1.46) and recurrent miscarriage (OR 3.5, 95% CI 1.03-12.01) compared to normal weight women (Lashen et al 2004). In women conceiving after assisted reproduction, the risks could be even higher.

A systematic review of the literature reported that women with BMI ≥25 who underwent assisted reproduction techniques, including IVF and intracytoplasmic sperm injection (ICSI), were more likely to miscarry than those of BMI <25 (OR 1.33, 95% CI 1.06-1.68). The risk was increased further in women with BMI ≥30 (OR 1.53, 95% CI 1.27-1.87). Women with BMI ≥ 25 had a lower pregnancy rate and required higher doses of gonadotrophins (Maheshwari et al 2007).

Hypertensive disorders

Obesity is well known to predispose to the development of hypertension in non pregnant individuals. A plethora of studies have demonstrated that obese women are also at increased risk of developing hypertensive disorders of pregnancy (HDP). Hypertensive disorders of pregnancy can include gestational hypertension, defined as new onset hypertension developing beyond 20 weeks of gestation, and pre eclampsia (PE), which is defined as new onset hypertension and proteinuria developing beyond 20 weeks gestation (Davey, MacGillivray 1988). The first and second trimester evaluation of risk (FASTER) trial prospectively examined rates of gestational hypertension and PE in 16 102 US women with BMI ≥30 and BMI ≥40 compared to those with BMI <30. Obese women were 2.5 times, and morbidly obese women 3.2 times, more likely to develop gestational hypertension than women of BMI <30 (Weiss et al 2004).

Similarly, obese and morbidly obese women were at greater risk of PE than women with BMI <30 (OR 1.6, 95% CI 1.1-2.25, and OR 3.3, 95% CI 2.4-4.4 respectively). A retrospective study of 24 241 primigravid women in Scotland reported equally strong associations between BMI and PE (Bhattacharya et al 2007). The report also revealed that in comparison with women of BMI 20-24.9, obese and morbidly obese women were at 3 and 7 times higher risk of PE respectively.

The 'dose dependent' relationship between maternal BMI and risk of PE was confirmed by a study of 1 174 women participating in a prospective cohort study of the pathogenesis of PE (Bodnar et al 2005). They observed a striking rise in the incidence of PE over the BMI range 15-30; compared with women of BMI 21, the risk of PE doubled at BMI 26 and tripled at BMI 30. Interestingly, this study also demonstrated substantial differences in risk of PE across the spectrum of normal BMI (18.5-24.9). For example, women with a BMI of 24 had a 70% greater risk of developing PE compared with women with BMI of 21. A strong protective effect of underweight was identified and this finding has been corroborated in at least two UK studies (Sebire et al 2001; Bhattacharya et al 2007).

Gestational diabetes

Gestational diabetes (GDM) is the clinical presentation of carbohydrate intolerance in pregnancy. The pathophysiology of GDM involves increased insulin resistance, which leads to reduced glucose uptake in muscle tissues and inadequate insulin response resulting in hyperglycaemia. Insulin resistance increases over the course of gestation in pregnant women of normal BMI but has been shown to be significantly greater in overweight and obese pregnant women (Catalano, Ehrenberg 2006). It is therefore unsurprising that obese pregnant women are at higher risk of developing GDM.

In the FASTER cohort, the incidence of GDM was reported at 2.3% for women with BMI <30, 6.3% for women with BMI ≥30 and 9.5% for women with BMI ≥40.

Based on this data the OR for the risk of GDM was 2.6 (95% CI 2.1-3.4) for obese and 4.0 (95% CI 3.1- 5.2) for morbidly obese women (Weiss et al 2004). The North West Thames Study also reported significantly increased risk of GDM among obese women (OR 3.6, 99% CI 3.25-3.98) (Sebire et al 2001). Although glycaemic control usually returns to normal following delivery, GDM is associated with an increased risk of developing type II diabetes in later life. The risk of developing type II diabetes following a pregnancy complicated by GDM is greatest in women who are overweight (O'Sullivan 1982).

Thromboembolism

A study by Greer (1994) found that normal pregnancy is associated with:
- Increased plasma concentrations of coagulation factors I, VII, VIII and X
- Decreased protein S
- Increased fibrinolysis
- Fivefold increase in the incidence of venous thrombosis.

Venous thrombosis and pulmonary embolism were identified as the leading cause of direct maternal death in the UK (Lewis 2007). A nested case control study using the Danish national birth registers reported an increased risk of venous thrombosis in both overweight and obese women compared to those with normal BMI (OR 1.4, 95% CI 0.7-2.8 and OR 5.3, 95% CI 2.1-13.5, respectively) (Larsen et al 2007).

Fetal risks

Congenital bnormalities

Maternal obesity has long been associated with an increased risk of congenital abnormalities (Waller et al 1994). A recent systematic review and meta analysis of 39 studies confirmed the association between maternal obesity and a wide range of structural fetal anomalies (Stothard et al 2009). Obesity increased the odds of the following congenital abnormalities:
- Neural tube defect (pooled OR 1.87, 95% CI 1.62-2.15)
- Spina bifida (OR 2.24, 95% CI 1.86-2.69)
- Cardiovascular anomalies (OR 1.3, 95% CI 1.12-1.51)
- Cleft lip and palate (OR 1.2, 95% CI 1.03-1.4)
- Anorectal atresia (OR 1.48, 95% CI 1.19-2.36)
- Limb reduction anomalies (OR 1.34, 95% CI 1.03-1.73).

However the risk of gastrochisis was significantly reduced among obese women.

The reasons for the increase in congenital abnormalities among obese women are not fully understood. One reason could be that ultrasound visualization of fetal anatomy is more difficult in obese pregnant women (Wolfe et al 1990). Decreased sensitivity of ultrasound for identifying abnormalities could result in fewer terminations and increased prevalence of defects at birth (Hendler et al 2004). However, Stothard et al (2009) reported no evidence of a decrease in OR in their analysis of studies which included data from terminations of pregnancy. Since obesity is a strong risk factor for diabetes, which is known to increase the risk of central nervous system and cardiovascular abnormalities (Towner et al 1995), it is possible that undiagnosed diabetes contributed to the increased incidence in obese women. Obesity is also associated with nutritional deficiencies such as notably reduced folate levels (Ray et al 2005). Therefore, folic acid supplementation at current levels may not offer the same protection against neural tube defects in obese women as for women of normal BMI.

Macrosomia

There is an increasing prevalence for obese women of macrosomia, also known as large for gestational age (LGA) babies. This is where the birthweight > 4 or > 4.5kg and birthweight > 90th centile for gestational age. Macrosomia is associated with a significant increase in maternal and perinatal morbidity. Analysis of data from the Danish Birth National Registers demonstrated an increase in numbers of newborns weighing > 4kg from 16.7% in 1990 to 20% in 1999 (Orskou et al 2001). The increasing prevalence of obesity among pregnant women has consistently been identified as an important factor underlying this trend; decreased maternal cigarette smoking and the increased incidence of diabetes in pregnancy are also potentially important. Baten et al (2001) studied 96 801 deliveries in Washington State US using multiple regression analysis to confirm an independent association between maternal obesity and birthweight >4kg. Furthermore, the risk of macrosomia was greater with each level of increase in BMI (BMI 20-24.9; OR 1.2, 95% CI 1.2-1.3, BMI 25-29.9; OR 1.5, 95% CI 1.4-1.6, BMI ≥30 OR 2.1, 95% CI 1.9-2.4). Eherenberg et al (2003) examined the relative contributions of diabetes and obesity to the prevalence of LGA in 12 950 pregnancies in Ohio US. Diabetes conferred the greatest risk of macrosomia (OR 4.4, 95% CI 2.9-6.7), compared to overweight (OR 1.2, 95% CI 1.1-1.4) and obesity (OR 1.6, 95% CI 1.4-1.9). However, the authors argued that increasing BMI is a more important contributor to the rising incidence of macrosomia in the population as a whole because of the lower prevalence of diabetes (5%) relative to overweight and obesity (47%). Moreover, the overweight and obese women in this study delivered 4 times more LGA infants than women with diabetes.

There is accumulating evidence that negative health impacts of macrosomia extend beyond the perinatal period. Being large at birth is increasingly associated with lifelong risks of poor health. Epidemiological studies, such as the US Nurses Health Study, reported a strong association between being large at birth and being overweight and obesity in adolescence and adulthood (Curhan et al 1996). Langer et al (2005) also reports that maternal obesity is also independently related to increased incidence of adolescent obesity. Children born to obese mothers have been shown to be twice as likely to be obese themselves by the age of 2 (15.1% with BMI > 95th centile for age) as children born to mothers of normal BMI (Whitaker 2004). Adolescent obesity is related to an increased risk of developing the metabolic syndrome; a clustering of clinical factors including hypertension, glucose intolerance and dyslipidaemia which markedly increase the risk of cardiovascular disease and diabetes. Furthermore, a recent study identified an increased hazard ratio for metabolic syndrome in children by age 11 who were either macrosomia at birth (2.19, 95% CI 1.25-3.82) or born to mothers with a prepregnancy BMI >27.5 (Boney et al 2005).

Intrauterine fetal death

Several large population-based studies suggest that maternal obesity is independently associated with an increased incidence of antepartum fetal death. A study of the Swedish National Birth Registers which included 167750 births, found the risk of late fetal death was observed to rise with increasing BMI even after adjusting for confounding factors. Compared with nulliparous women with a BMI <20, the adjusted risk for antepartum stillbirth doubled in nulliparous women with normal BMI (20-24.9), tripled in overweight nulliparous women (BMI 25-29.5), and quadrupled in nulliparous women with BMI ≥30 (Cnattingus et al 1998). In parous women, only obesity increased risk of late fetal death (OR 2.0, 95% CI 1.2-3.3). Notably, weight gain during pregnancy was not associated with any increase in antepartum fetal death. This data was supported by a Danish study of 24505 singleton pregnancies which found obesity was associated with a doubled risk of stillbirth (OR 2.8, 95% CI 1.5-5.3) and neonatal death (OR 2.6, 95% CI 1.2-5.8), compared to normal weight women (Kristensen et al 2005). Furthermore, a study of 54505 pregnancies within the Danish Birth Registers demonstrated that the incidence of fetal death increased with advancing gestational age. Compared with normal weight women, the hazard ratio (HR) for fetal death in obese women was 2.1 (95% CI 1.0-4.4) from 28-36 weeks, 3.5 (95% CI 1.9-6.4) at 37-39 weeks gestation and 4.6 (95% CI 1.6-13.4) at 40+ weeks (Nohr et al 2005). The median birth weights reported for the unexplained deaths in obese women were lower than the median birthweight for the live birth group. This finding suggests intrauterine growth restriction might have contributed to the increased death rate in this study.

The North West Thames study demonstrated a more modest increase in risk of intrauterine death in obese women (OR 1.4, 95% CI 1.1-1.7), after adjusting for obesity related complications of pregnancy (Sebire et al 2001). However, the

Aberdeen cohort study (Bhattacharya et al 2007) recently reported a significant increase in risk of stillbirth in obese women (OR 1.8, CI 1.1-2.9). The stillbirth rate has remained around 5 per 1000 births in the UK for the last decade, after years of steady decline since the 1950s. It is possible that increase in obesity among pregnant women has contributed to this lack of improvement but further studies will be necessary to establish whether this is the case.

Intrapartum and post partum risks

In addition to the increased risk of antenatal and fetal problems, obese women are more likely to experience complications and medical intervention in the peripartum period.

Preterm birth

Most studies report low prepregnancy BMI and poor gestational weight gain as the strongest risk factors for preterm delivery (Schieve et al 1999). The data regarding the risk in obese women is conflicting with reports of increased (Baeten et al 2001), decreased (Sebire et al 2001) and unchanged (Jensen et al 2003) rates of preterm delivery compared to normal weight women. Current evidence suggests that obesity may increase the rate of iatrogenic preterm birth, indicated due to obstetric or maternal medical conditions (which account for up to 25% of all preterm deliveries) rather than spontaneous preterm delivery (Nohr et al 2007).

Caesarean section (CS)

A recent meta analysis of 11 studies from 1996-2007 demonstrated that the risk of caesarean delivery in nulliparous singleton pregnancies is increased 1.5 times in overweight (BMI 25-30), 2.25 times in obese (BMI 30-35) and 3.36 times in severely obese (BMI ≥35) women compared to women with BMI of 20-25, even when controlling for other factors (Poobalan et al 2009). The authors also identified a slightly increased risk of emergency compared to elective caesarean delivery in the subset of studies which examined rates of emergency caesarean. This increased risk is a serious concern; caesarean delivery in an obese woman may be more technically challenging because of the increased risks of anaesthesia (Saravanakumar et al 2006) and operative complications such as excessive bleeding (Catalano 2007). Caesarean section is associated with an increased risk of postoperative complications, such as wound infection and deep vein thrombosis, due to prolonged immobilization.

The reasons why obese women are at greater risk of caesarean delivery is unclear. A recent study of the Swedish National Birth Registers found that obesity in the first trimester of pregnancy was associated with greater likelihood of postdates pregnancies and a lower incidence of spontaneous onset of labour at term compared with normal weight women (BMI 20-25) (Denison et al 2008). The proportion of women with BMI ≥35 who went into spontaneous labour at term was 50% lower than of those with a normal BMI in the first trimester. Postdates pregnancy are associated with increased obstetric intervention including induction of labour, epidural anaesthesia and use of oxytocin (Heslehurst et al 2008), which in turn leads to higher risk of operative vaginal delivery and CS.

Postpartum risks

In addition to the peripartum risks outlined above, overweight and obese women are also at increased risk of postnatal wound, genital and urinary tract infections compared to those of normal BMI (Heslehurst et al 2008). Increased morbidity, including higher rates of thromboembolism and postpartum haemorrhage, may explain the increased duration of hospitalization observed in obese women. A recent meta-analysis of 49 studies worldwide reported that women of normal BMI stayed in hospital for 2-3 days, overweight and obese women for 2-4 days and morbidly obese women for 3-5 days. Neonatal unit admission was also increased for infants of obese women (Heslehurst et al 2008).

Several studies both in European and US women suggest that obesity negatively affects breastfeeding. A high prepregnancy BMI is associated with reduced initiation (Oddy et al 2006) and shorter duration of full or any breastfeeding (Baker et al 2007). The mechanisms underlying this relationship require further examination but obesity is associated with a reduction in the prolactin response to suckling in the first postnatal week and a delay in the onset of copious milk secretion (Hilson et al 2004; Rasmussen and Kjolhede 2004).

Conclusion

An increasing proportion of women in the UK are obese at the start of pregnancy and this trend shows no signs of slowing. Obesity alone confers an increased risk of poor health including cancer, diabetes and cardiovascular disease and is a serious threat to public health. Maternal prepregnancy obesity is a significant risk factor for poor maternal and fetal outcomes in pregnancy and the effects may impact on long term health. Improving outcomes for obese pregnant women and their babies presents an important challenge to healthcare.

The ideal goal would be for obese women to lose weight through diet and lifestyle changes before conception. However this may not be realistic as achieving and maintaining weight loss is recognised to be difficult and many pregnancies are unplanned. Improving awareness of the specific effects of obesity on pregnancy outcome among the general public is necessary. Weight loss during pregnancy is not advised because of the potential for negative effects on fetal growth. Limiting weight gain may reduce the risk of complications, but a full evaluation of benefits and potential harms of recommended weight gain targets is necessary to determine unexpected consequences which could impact on fetal development and future health.

Preliminary studies have shown that increased physical activity improves outcomes in sedentary pregnant women and might benefit women who are obese. Large trials are needed to determine the efficacy and acceptability of exercise programmes for obese pregnant women.

References

Baeten JM, Bukusi EA, Lambe M (2001) Pregnancy complications and outcomes among overweight and obese nulliparous women. *Am J Public Health* **91**: 436–40.

Baker JL, Michaelsen KF, Sorensen TI *et al* (2007) High prepregnant body mass index is associated with early termination of full and any breastfeeding in Danish women. *Am J Clin Nutr* **86**: 404–11

Bhattacharya S, Campbell DM, Liston, WA (2007) Effect of Body Mass Index on pregnancy outcomes in nulliparous women delivering singleton babies. *BMC Public Health* **7**: 168.

Bodnar LM, Ness RB, Markovic N *et al* (2005) The risk of preeclampsia rises with increasing prepregnancy body mass index. *Ann Epidemiol* **15**: 475–82.

Boney CM, Verma A, Tucker R *et al* (2005) Metabolic syndrome in childhood: association with birth weight, maternal obesity, and gestational diabetes mellitus. *Pediatrics* **115**: e290–6.

Catalano PM (2007) Management of obesity in pregnancy. *Obstet Gynecol* **109**: 419–33.

Catalano, PM, Ehrenberg HM (2006) The short- and long-term implications of maternal obesity on the mother and her offspring. *BJOG* **113**: 1126–33.

Cnattingus, S, Bergstrom, R, Lipworth, L et al (1998) Prepregnancy weight and the risk of adverse outcomes. N Engl J Med 338(3):147-52.

Confidential Enquiry into Maternal and Child Health (2007) *Perinatal Mortality 2005: England, Wales and Northern Ireland*. CEMACH, London.

Curhan GC, Chertow GM, Willett WC *et al* (1996) Birth weight and adult hypertension and obesity in women. *Circulation* **94**: 1310–5.

Davey DA, MacGillivray I (1988) The classification and definition of the hypertensive disorders of pregnancy. *Am J Obstet Gynecol* **158**: 892–8.

Denison FC, Price J, Graham C *et al* (2008). Maternal obesity, length of gestation, risk of postdates pregnancy and spontaneous onset of labour at term. *BJOG* **115**: 720–5.

Department of Health, (2004) National Centre for Social Research, Department of Epidemiology and Public Health at the Royal Free and University College Medical School *Health Survey for England 2003*. London

Ehrenberg HM, Huston-Presley L, Catalano PM (2003) The influence of obesity and gestational diabetes mellitus on accretion and the distribution of adipose tissue in pregnancy. *Am J Obstet Gynecol* **189**: 944–8.

Foresight (2007) *Tackling Obesities: Future Choices - Project Report*. Government Office for Science, London.

Forouhi NG, Sattar N (2006) CVD risk factors and ethnicity--a homogeneous relationship? *Atheroscler Suppl*, **7**: 11–9.

Greer IA (1994) Haemostasis and thrombosis in pregnancy. In *Haemostasis and thrombosis in pregnancy* (Eds, Bloom A L, Forbes CD, Thomas DP and Tuddenham EGD) Churchill Livingstone, Edinburgh: 987–1015.

Guo SS, Wu W, Chumlea WC *et al* (2002) Predicting overweight and obesity in adulthood from body mass index values in childhood and adolescence. *Am J Clin Nutr* **76**: 653–8.

Hendler I, Blackwell SC, Bujold E *et al* (2004) The impact of maternal obesity on midtrimester sonographic visualization of fetal cardiac and craniospinal structures. *Int J Obes Relat Metab Disord* **28**: 1607–11.

Heslehurst N, Ells LJ, Simpson H, *et al* (2007) Trends in maternal obesity incidence rates, demographic predictors, and health inequalities in 36,821 women over a 15-year period. *BJOG* **114**: 187–94.

Heslehurst N, Simpson H, Ells LJ *et al* (2008) The impact of maternal BMI status on pregnancy outcomes with immediate short-term obstetric resource implications: a meta-analysis. *Obes Rev* **9**(6):635-83

Hilson JA, Rasmussen KM, Kjolhede CL (2004) High prepregnant body mass index is associated with poor lactation outcomes among white, rural women independent of psychosocial and demographic correlates. *J Hum Lact* **20**: 18–29.

Institute of Medicine (1990) Nutritional status and weight gain. In *Nutrition During Pregnancy*. National Academies Press, Washington DC: 27–233.

Jensen DM, Damm P, Sorensen B*et al* (2003) Pregnancy outcome and prepregnancy body mass index in 2459 glucose-tolerant Danish women. *Am J Obstet Gynecol* **189**: 239–44.

Kanagalingam MG, Forouhi NG, Greer IA *et al* (2005) Changes in booking body mass index over a decade: retrospective analysis from a Glasgow Maternity Hospital. *BJOG* **112**: 1431–3.

Kinoshita T, Itoh M (2006) Longitudinal variance of fat mass deposition during pregnancy evaluated by ultrasonography: the ratio of visceral fat to subcutaneous fat in the abdomen. *Gynecol Obstet Invest* **61**: 115–8.

Klein S, Allison DB, Heymsfield SB et al (2007) Waist circumference and cardiometabolic risk: a consensus statement from Shaping America's Health: Association for Weight Management and Obesity Prevention; NAASO, The Obesity Society; the American Society for Nutrition; and the American Diabetes Association. *Am J Clin Nutr* **85**,:1197–202.

Langer O, Yogev Y, Xenakis EM *et al* (2005) Overweight and obese in gestational diabetes: the impact on pregnancy outcome. *Am J Obstet Gynecol* **192**: 1768–76.

Larsen TB, Sorensen HT, Gislum M, *et al* (2007) Maternal smoking, obesity, and risk of venous thromboembolism during pregnancy and the puerperium: a population-based nested case-control study. *Thromb Res* **120**: 505–9.

Lashen H, Fear K, Sturdee DW (2004) Obesity is associated with increased risk of first trimester and recurrent miscarriage: matched case-control study. *Hum Reprod* **19**:1644–6.

Lewis G, Drife J (2004) *The Confidential Enquiry into Maternal and Child Health: Why Mothers Die 2000-2002. The Sixth Report of the Confidential Enquiries into Maternal Deaths in the United Kingdom.*, RCOG London.

Lewis GE (2007) *The Confidential Enquiry into Maternal and Child Health (CEMACH): Saving Mothers' Lives; reviewing maternal deaths to make motherhood safer 2003-2005. The Seventh Report on the Confidential Enquiries into Maternal Deaths in the United Kingdom*, CEMACH London.

Maheshwari A, Stofberg L, Bhattacharya S (2007) Effect of overweight and obesity on assisted reproductive technology--a systematic review. *Hum Reprod Update* **13**: 433–44.

Malik VS, Schulze MB, Hu FB (2006) Intake of sugar-sweetened beverages and weight gain: a systematic review. *Am J Clin Nutr* **84**: 274–88.

Mukhopadhyay B, Forouhi NG, FisherBM *et al* (2006) A comparison of glycaemic and metabolic control over time among South Asian and European patients with Type 2 diabetes: results from follow-up in a routine diabetes clinic. *Diabet Med* **23**: 94–8.

Must A, Spadano J, Coakley EH *et al* (1999) The disease burden associated with overweight and obesity. *JAMA* **282**: 1523–9.

NICE (2008) *Antenatal Care: Routine Care for the Healthy Pregnant Woman*, National Institute for Health and Clinical Excellence, London.

Nohr, EA, Bech, BH, Davies, MJ et al (2005) Prepregnancy obesity and fetal death: A study within the Danish National Birth Cohort. *Obstet Gynecol* **106**(2): 250-9.

Nohr, EA, Bech, BH, Vaeth, M et al (2007) Obesity, gestational weight gain and preterm birth: A study within the Danish National Birth Cohort. *Paediatr Perinat Epidemiol* **21**(1): 5-14.

Oddy WH, Li J, Landsborough L *et al* (2006) The association of maternal overweight and obesity with breastfeeding duration. *J Pediatr* **149**: 185–91.

O'Rahilly S, Farooqi IS, Yeo, GS *et al* (2003) Minireview: human obesity-lessons from monogenic disorders. *Endocrinology* **144**: 3757–64.

Orskou J, Kesmodel U, Henriksen TB *et al* (2001) An increasing proportion of infants weigh more than 4000 grams at birth. *Acta Obstet Gynecol Scand* **80**: 931–6.

O'Sullivan JB (1982) Body weight and subsequent diabetes mellitus. *JAMA* **248**: 949–52.

Pereira MA, Kartashov AI, Ebbeling CB *et al* (2005) Fast-food habits, weight gain, and insulin resistance (the CARDIA study): 15-year prospective analysis. *Lancet* **365**: 36–42.

Pietilainen KH, Rissanen A, Laamanen M *et al* (2004) Growth patterns in young adult monozygotic twin pairs discordant and concordant for obesity. *Twin Res* **7**: 421–9.

Poobalan AS, Aucott LS, Gurung T *et al* (2009) Obesity as an independent risk factor for elective and emergency caesarean delivery in nulliparous women--systematic review and meta-analysis of cohort studies. *Obes Rev* **10**: 28–35.

Rasmussen KM, Kjolhede CL (2004) Prepregnant overweight and obesity diminish the prolactin response to suckling in the first week postpartum. *Pediatrics* **113**: e465–71.

Ray JG, Wyatt PR, Vermeulen MJ *et al* (2005) Greater maternal weight and the ongoing risk of neural tube defects after folic acid flour fortification. *Obstet Gynecol* **105**:261–5.

Saravanakumar K, Rao SG, Cooper, GM (2006) Obesity and obstetric anaesthesia. *Anaesthesia* **61**: 36–48.

Schieve LA, Cogswell ME, Scanlon, KS (1999) Maternal weight gain and preterm delivery: differential effects by body mass index. *Epidemiology* **10**: 141–7.

Sebire NJ, Jolly M, Harris JP *et al* (2001) Maternal obesity and pregnancy outcome: a study of 287,213 pregnancies in London. *Int J Obes Relat Metab Disord* **25**: 1175–82.

Shen W, Punyanitya M, Chen J *et al* (2006) Waist circumference correlates with metabolic syndrome indicators better than percentage fat. *Obesity (Silver Spring)* **14**: 727–36.

Stothard KJ, Tennant PW, Bell R *et al* (2009) Maternal overweight and obesity and the risk of congenital anomalies: a systematic review and meta-analysis. *JAMA* **301**: 636–50.

The NHS Information Centre (2009) *Statistics on obesity, physical activity and diet: England, February 2009*, London.

Towner D, Kjos SL, Leung B *et al* (1995) Congenital malformations in pregnancies complicated by NIDDM. *Diabetes Care* **18**: 1446–51.

Usha Kiran TS, Hemmadi S, Bethel J *et al* (2005) Outcome of pregnancy in a woman with an increased body mass index. *BJOG* **112**: 768–72.

Waller DK, Mills JL., Simpson JL *et al* (1994) Are obese women at higher risk for producing malformed offspring? *Am J Obstet Gynecol* **170**: 541–8.

Wardle J, Brodersen NH, Cole T. J *et al* (2006) Development of adiposity in adolescence: five year longitudinal study of an ethnically and socioeconomically diverse sample of young people in Britain. *BMJ* **332**: 1130–5.

Weiss JL, Malone FD, Emig D *et al* (2004) Obesity, obstetric complications and cesarean delivery rate--a population-based screening study. *Am J Obstet Gynecol* **190**: 1091–7.

Whitaker RC (2004) Predicting preschooler obesity at birth: the role of maternal obesity in early pregnancy. *Pediatrics* **114**: e29–36.

WHO (1997) *Obesity: Preventing and managing the global epidemic: Report of a WHO Consultation on Obesity*, World Health Organization Geneva.

WHO Expert Consultation (2004) Appropriate body mass index for Asian populations and its implication for policy and intervention strategies. *Lancet* **363**: 157–163.

Wolfe HM, Sokol RJ, Martier SM *et al* (1990) Maternal obesity: a potential source of error in sonographic prenatal diagnosis. *Obstet Gynecol* **76**: 339–42.

Yusuf S, Hawken S, Ounpuu S *et al* (2005) Obesity and the risk of myocardial infarction in 27,000 participants from 52 countries: a case-control study. *Lancet*, **366**, 1640-9 myocardial infarction in 27,000 participants from 52 countries: a case-control study. *Lancet* **366**: 1640–9.

Chapter 2

Bariatric Surgery and Care of Pregnant Women

Yana Richens and Alberic Fiennes

Introduction

As the obesity epidemic continues to rise, midwives are going to be faced with new clinical challenges, one of these being the care and management of women who have undergone bariatric surgery.

In the United States the incidence of bariatric surgery increased by 800% between 1998 and 2005 (from 12480 to 113500 cases). Women accounted for 83% of procedures in the 18 to 45-year age group (Maggard et al 2009).

The picture is similar in the United Kingdom; the number of adults and children undergoing bariatirc surgery in the National Health Service increased by 40%. In 2007/2008 this number was 2724, an increase of 40% since the previous year (1951 in 2006/07). Of this group, 598 were males and 2126 females (Information Centre for Health and Social Care 2009). However this figure does not include the number of private operations. One private hospital group reported that 12848 people sought surgery last year which is 74% higher than the previous year (Martin 2009).

The aim of the article is to highlight the differences of the types of surgery and the midwife's role in supporting this group of women.

The term "bariatric surgery" is an umbrella term often used to define a group of procedures that can be performed to facilitate weight loss. This term is preferred over "obesity surgery", because patients may perceive a stigma in the term "obese". It includes gastric bands, "gastroplasties" (these are various "staplings"), stomach stapling, gastric bypasses, sleeve gastrectomy and biliopancreatic diversion. This surgery is used in the treatment of obesity for people with a Body Mass Index (BMI) above 40 or for people with a BMI between 35 and 40 who have health problems, for example Type 2 diabetes or heart disease. Comparing surgery with non operative surgery, the National Institute for Health and Clinical Excellence (NICE 2006) analysed the evidence and concluded: "Surgery remains more effective than a non-surgical approach for people who are obese (BMI $\geq$38 kg/m2 for women, $\geq$

34 for men) in the longer term (measured up to 10 years after surgery)". See *Box 1* for current advice provided by NICE (2006).

The first thing you as a midwife will need to know is the type of surgery that a woman has undergone. This is essential as some procedures are reversible and only mechanically restrict the amount of food that a woman can eat, whereas other procedures are more permanent and will affect absorption of nutrients. This group of women will require a team approach to care during the pregnancy. As well as the midwife, this includes a bariatric surgeon, an obstetrician and a specialist dietician and/or nurse specialist. Many of these women may, initially, know more about their dietary requirements than their obstetrician or midwife and will be taking vitamin supplements prescribed by their bariatric teams.

Box 1

- Bariatric surgery is recommended as a treatment option for adults with obesity if all of the following criteria are fulfilled:
  - they have a BMI of 40 kg/m2 or more, or between 35 kg/m2 and 40 kg/m2 and other significant disease (for example, type 2 diabetes or high blood pressure) that could be improved if they lost weight
  - all appropriate non-surgical measures have been tried but have failed to achieve or maintain adequate, clinically beneficial weight loss for at least 6 months
  - the person has been receiving or will receive intensive management in a specialist obesity service
  - the person is generally fit for anaesthesia and surgery
  - the person commits to the need for long-term follow-up.
- Bariatric surgery is also recommended as a first-line option (instead of lifestyle interventions or drug treatment) for adults with a BMI of more than 50 kg/m2 in whom surgical intervention is considered appropriate.

Types of procedures

Gastric band

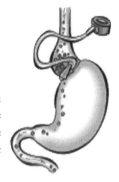

Laparoscopic Adjustable Gastric Banding (LAGB)

The gastric band is implanted laparoscopically, which usually takes around 30-45 minutes. Although adjustable bands were first fitted in the mid 1980s, the procedure became popular after the first human laparoscopic procedure in Belgium in 1993.

How it works

This is a purely restrictive and more or less reversible surgical procedure. It works by restricting food intake, creating a small upper-stomach pouch that mechanically limits food intake capacity. The feeling of fullness after meals is often absent. This procedure does not affect absorption. A silicone band is placed around the upper part of the stomach and moulds the stomach into two connected chambers. The band has a tubular balloon on its inner surface, and when this is inflated with liquid (by injection into a sub-cutaneous port), the band is tightened. The mechanical restriction to food intake increases and less is consumed at any one time. The concept that the brain would be "tricked" into feeling that the whole stomach is full has more recently been shown to be theoretically wrong and it may not occur in practice. Nevertheless, many patients do get a good weight loss result.

Overall calorie intake may be 50-60% less than usual, leading to weight loss. As the food is slowly digested in the pouch, it passes through the band stoma (opening) into the normal stomach below.

Food digestion occurs through the normal digestive process, and there is no selective effect on intake beyond personal food choices. The latter may nevertheless lead to micronutrient (e.g. iron) deficiency.

The key during pregnancy is to remember that the band is adjustable and can be deflated during pregnancy. Deflation of the band may be required during the first trimester due to nausea and vomiting. This will enable a higher intake of food. Some women may have difficulty in swallowing medication and it maybe a good idea to think about liquid vitamins. Heartburn may also be excessive, and this may be relieved by deflating the gastric band, once again threatening weight regain. For this reason women may resist deflation. Deflation is advisable shortly before expected delivery. Women who have undergone gastric band surgery will have the same nutritional requirements as women who have not had a gastric band, however this will be different for women who have undergone other forms of surgery.

Gastric Bypass

Restrictive and "malabsorptive" procedures

Gastric Bypass is also know as "Roux-en-Y" gastric bypass (RYGBP) after the Swiss surgeon César Roux (1857-1934) who devised the method of diverting food away from an excluded stomach during the treatment of cancers and ulcers. This operation leads to, and sustains, long-term weight loss by a combination of restriction and other mechanisms. Traditionally it is regarded as a combination of restriction and mal-absorption.

How it works

In this procedure, a small stomach pouch is created, which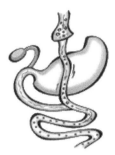
is separated off from the rest of the stomach. The pouch
has a volume of 20-40 ml and is severely restrictive, at
least at the outset. The outlet from this newly formed
pouch empties directly into the mid-portion of the
jejunum, thus bypassing the first 50-100 cms completely.
Also, in this "Roux loop" food is delayed in mixing
with bile and the pancreatic juices that aid in the absorption of nutrients.
However, the evidence that the actual amount of intestine excluded results
in significant calorie mal-adsorption is scanty. Patients who had the same
amount of intestine excluded for other reasons frequently have no weight
loss and attempts to "tailor" the intestinal limb lengths have not worked. The
faeces do contain increased fat, but not greatly so. There clearly is however
another powerful effect, because patients do experience profound early
satiety (feeling of fullness) and often a complete loss of appetite and food
cravings. This is now known to be due to enhanced release of the intestinal
hormone Peptide YY-36 ("PYY"), which is a natural appetite suppressant
and glucose metabolism regulator.

Although there is little evidence for calorie mal-adsorption, there are
nevertheless important micronutrient effects. Stomach acid is excluded
and dietary ferric iron is no longer reduced to absorbable ferrous iron.
Vitamin B12 absorption may be affected. The duodenal exclusion
profoundly affects calcium absorption and it is traditional to give high-
dose 25-OH-vitamin D and calcium supplements. Note that the morbidly
obese population may be moderately vitamin D deficient before surgery.
By contrast, concerns about vitamin A deficiency are based historically
on other kinds of surgery. The commonest cause of a low vitamin A level
is sample processing, and in view of its potential toxicity it may be not
be useful to give supplements.

Mal-absorptive procedures

Biliopancreatic Diversion (BPD)
This procedure was developed by Professor Nicola Scopinaro in Italy and
was introduced in 1979. It combines the benefits of restriction and mal-
absorption. Part of the stomach is resected however the patient can eat a free
diet as this does not cause major mechanical restriction. The distal part of
the small intestine is then connected to the remaining stomach, bypassing the
duodenum and jejunum.

How it works

Biliopancreatic diversion is a truly calorie mal-adsorptive procedure. In its original form, partial removal of the stomach was undertaken not with restrictive intent – which would indeed run the risk of protein-calorie deficiency – but as a means of preventing peptic ulceration at the gastro-intestinal anastomosis, in the era before proton pump inhibitors. In derivatives of BPD, mild stomach-restrictive surgery (sleeve gastrectomy) is undertaken. The small intestine is then divided with one end attached to the stomach pouch to create what is called an "alimentary limb." All the food moves through this segment, however not much is absorbed. The bile and pancreatic juices necessary for digestion move through the "biliopancreatic limb," which is connected to the side of the intestine close to the end. This supplies digestive juices in the section of the intestine now called the "common channel". Because the food only mixes with the biliopancreatic juices necessary for digestion at a late stage, fats and carbohydrates are permanently mal-absorbed. The surgeon is able to vary the length of the common limb to regulate the limiting amount of absorption of carbohydrate, fat, and fat-soluble vitamins that can be absorbed. Protein can be absorbed by mass effect and is absorbed even in the ascending colon, but this cannot greatly affect calorie intake.

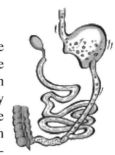

Pregnancy after bariatric surgery

Recent evidence suggests that becoming pregnant after bariatric surgery is actually less risky than becoming pregnant while still obese. A systematic review of 75 studies found that rates of adverse outcomes for pregnant women and newborn babies may be lower after bariatric surgery, when compared with pregnant women who are still obese (Maggard et al 2008). The findings of the review concluded that none of the women who had bariatric surgery in these studies developed gestational diabetes, compared with 22.1% of obese women did develop gestational diabetes. In addition, none of the pregnant women who had weight loss surgery developed PE, compared with 3.1% of women who were obese during pregnancy.

Women who had bariatric surgery also gained less weight during their pregnancy than those who did not have surgery.

Two very early studies by Martin (1988) and Haddow (1988) reported a higher than expected number of neural tube defects in babies born to women who had bariatric surgery. It was reported that mothers at risk were those who did not take the recommended vitamin supplements. Generally newborn outcomes were similar or better after surgery compared with obese women without laparoscopic adjustable gastric band surgery (7.7% vs. 7.1% for premature delivery; 7.7% vs. 10.6% for low birth weight; 7.7% vs. 14.6% for macrosomia.

A most recent case-controlled study by Wax et al (2009) reported no difference in obstetric outcome, whether conception was early (<18 months) or late after RYGBP. Nevertheless it is traditional to firmly advise reliable contraception for a year after RYGBP and BPD. As there are no reliable studies on the absorption of the oral contraceptive, it should not be regarded as "reliable". Therefore condoms should be used.

Surgical complications in pregnancies following bariatric surgery

The sytematic review by Maggard et al (2008) identifed 20 reported complications which required surgical intervention during pregnancy. The majority of these women complained of pain, at first thought to be non specific abdominal pain. This pain occurred from 13 to 37 weeks gestation. If any woman who has undergone bariatric surgery reports this symptom to a midwife, it is essential it is taken very seriously and discussed with both obstetricians and bariatric surgeon. The reported complications included 14 bowel obstructions (11 internal hernias), one gastric ulcer, four band problems and a staple line stricture. Given reporting bias and the very high incidence of gastric bypass (>150000 operations world-wide last year), however these complications may be no more common than in the non-pregnant population. Midwives need to be aware of them when symptoms are reported and take appropriate action.

Care of the woman and baby: the role of the midwife

Currently there is a dearth of literature on how midwives should care for this group of women. The major concern by midwives when providing antenatal care for this group of women will be micro-nutritional deficiences. Deficiencies in iron, vitamin A, vitamin B_{12}, vitamin K, folate and calcium can result in both maternal complications, such as severe anaemia, and fetal complications, such as congenital abnormalities, decreased IUGR and failure to thrive. However in reality it is rarely an actual problem In women taking correct supplements these concerns are not often justified and are readily allayed by routine antenatal blood tests. Often this group of women will also need increased psychological care. This can be for two reasons: firstly they have concerns about the growing baby and "is the baby receiving the right amount of nutrients?". The available evidence supports a cautiously reassuring stance. In our own experience fetal growth tends to proceed normally even in women actively losing weight. Occasionally this fear may be fuelled by nagging "guilt" that a woman has somehow harmed her future baby by being so "weak" as to need bariatric surgery. It is clearly professionally correct to be very firm in the position that, on the contrary, the woman has courageously taken a life-altering step which has enhanced the future health prospects of her child. Secondly, women who suffered from morbid obesity occasionally had at the outset or later develop a disordered body image. As the pregnancy progresses their body shape will change and old fears may return. As these may in turn fuel the resurgence of an eating disorder, it is advsiable to provide constant reassurance and support, as well as to be alert to the potential need for intervention.

Women who have undergone a gastric bypass should have been prescribed a micronutrient replacement by their bariatric surgeon. Although this normally includes Pregaday, and thus folic acid, as a midwife you must ensure that the woman understands the importance of this and is actively taking the correct medication. Some women will also be very anxious about the dose of vitamin A that they may be taking, as this is often present in the supplementation. With standard proprietary multivitamin preparations such as Forceval or Sanatogen Gold, toxicity is extremely unlikely, unless a falsely low Vitamin A level has been misinterpreted, leading to parenteral supplementation. However, vitamin A deficiency and a genuine need for major supplements may occur after truly mal-adsorptive procedures such as BPD. In any case of doubt, a correctly taken and processed plasma vitamin A level may give the woman reassurance.

Early booking is essential for this group of women, normal antenatal booking bloods should be taken and in addition a standard bypass/BPD micronutrient screen, as routinely advised at least yearly after these procedures. This includes serum iron/TIBC; vitamin B12/folate; 25-OH-vitamin D; Vitamin A; bone profile; urea, electrolytes and creatinine; LFTs. Magnesium, Zinc and Copper are also measured in some bariatric units. It may be prudent to recheck all these, at least during rapid fetal growth. Since pouch outlet stricture or an overtight band may lead to additional vomiting, vitamin B6 estimation is prudent in such cases.

A normal delivery should be advised. It may be advisable to somewhat loosen a gastric band a week or two before anticipated delivery.

Providing safe effective care for this group of pregnant women will be challenging for midwives and for the team involved in meeting the needs of both the woman and her family. At the present time there is no national guidance or evidence based guideline on how to achieve this, however the authors would suggest that this can be achieved by good communication between professional by planning and involving the woman in her own care. Above all midwives will need to listen carefully to the women at each antenatal consultation.

References

Cedergren MI (2004). Maternal morbid obesity and the risk of adverse pregnancy outcome. *Obstetrics & Gynecology* **103**(2): 219–24

CEMACH (2007) Saving Mothers Lives 2003-2005 A report of the UK confidential enquiries into maternal deaths

CEMACH (2004) Confidential Enquiry into Maternal and Child Health. Why Mothers Die 2002-2004. The Sixth Report

Chu SY, Kim SY et al (2007). Maternal obesity and risk of caesarean delivery: a meta-analysis. *Obesity Reviews* **8**(5): 385–94

Haddow JE, Hill LE, Kloza EM et al (1986) Neural tube defects after gastric bypass. *Lancet* **1**(8493): 1330

Information Centre for Health and Social Care (2009) Statistics on obesity, physical activity and diet: England, accessed 16th April 2009 http://www.ic.nhs.uk/webfiles/publications/opan09/OPAD%20Feb%202009%20final.pdf

Jevitt C, Hernadex MS, Groer M (2007) Lactation Complicated by Overweight and Obesity: Supporting the Mother and Newborn. *Journal of Midwifery and Women's Health* **52**(6): 607–13

National Institute for Health and Clinical Excellence (NICE) (2006) Clinical Guideline No.43. Obesity: guidance on the prevention, identification, assessment and management of overweight and obesity in adults and children. Evidence table Section 5, 15.3.5; 638

Maggard, MD, Irina Yermilov, Zhaoping Li, et al (2008) Pregnancy and Fertility Following Bariatric Surgery: A Systematic Review. *JAMA* **300**: 2286–96

Martin D (2009) How the Fern effect has given a boost to gastric band surgery *Daily Mail* **17.04.2009:** 36

Martin L, Chavez GF, Adams MJ Jr et al 1988 Gastric bypass surgery as maternal risk factor for neural tube defects. *Lancet* **1**(8586): 640–1

Richens Y (2008) Tackling Maternal Obesity: Suggestions for midwives. *British Journal of Midwifery* **16**(1): 14–9

Sebire NJ, Jolly M, Harris JP, et al (2001) Maternal obesity and pregnancy outcome: a study of 287,213 pregnancies in London. *Int J Obes Relat Metab Disord* **25**: 1175–82

Usha Kiran TS, Hemmadi S et al (2005) Outcome of pregnancy in a woman with an increased body mass index. *BJOG* **112**(6): 768–72

Wax JR, Cartin A, Wolff R et al (2009) Pregnancy following Gastric Bypass Surgery for Morbid Obesity: Effect of Surgery-to-Conception Interval on Maternal and Neonatal Outcomes. *Obes Surg* **18:** 1517–21

Weiss JL, Malone FD, Emig D et al (2004) Obesity, obstetric complications and cesarean delivery rate – a population based screening study. *Am J Obstet Gynecol* **190:** 1091–7

Chapter 3

Ultrasonography and the Obese Woman

Pranav Pandya and Julie Hogg

Introduction

The prevalence of obesity, defined as a body mass index (BMI) of >30, has significantly increased during the last three decades. The Department of Health (DH) (2002) reported that 32% of women aged 35-64 years in England are obese and has predicted that if current trends continue, six million women will be obese by 2010. There are significant health implications of prepregnancy maternal obesity for the woman and baby. From an obstetric ultrasound perspective these include miscarriage, congenital structural malformations, hypertensive disorders, fetal macrosomia, intrauterine growth restriction and prolonged pregnancy. All of which result in an increased risk of perinatal morbidity and mortality. This is compounded by the fact that there are technical difficulties in obtaining appropriate views because of maternal habitus. In addition there is an increased prevalence of repetitive strain injury (RSI) in sonographers who have to routinely scan these women.

This chapter will focus on the role of prenatal ultrasound to diagnose and manage these complications and discuss the limitations of obstetric ultrasound in this group of women.

Specific considerations in prenatal ultrasound of obese women

Ultrasound imaging of the obese patient is challenging due to the adverse effects of obesity on sound waves. Image clarity increases with ultrasound frequency, however tissue penetration decreases with increasing frequency. Therefore in obese women, lower frequency transducers are required which compromises the clarity of images. The intensity of an ultrasound beam is attenuated as it passes through tissue which is exaggerated in the imaging of the obese woman. Excess subcutaneous adiposity and increased connective tissue result in poor image quality (*Figure 3.1*). It is however important to note that body mass index (BMI) alone is not useful in predicting the difficulties encountered with ultrasound visualisation because abdominal adiposity is the main issue with obstetric imaging.

Wolfe et al (1990) reported a 14.5% fall in visualisation of fetal structures in women with increased BMI. In addition, Wong et al (2002) studied the connection between diabetes, obesity and sonographic visualisation. The image quality was considered to be unsatisfactory in 37% of diabetic women and this study concluded that this high rate was mainly due to increased BMI in the diabetes group. They noted that there was not only a high incidence of incomplete and sub-optimal first examinations but also that the majority of women who had repeat ultrasound examinations still had sub-optimal views (86%).

It is therefore essential that sonographers, midwives and doctors performing ultrasound examinations know how to optimise views of the fetal structures. This will include utilising an appropriate ultrasound machine that complies with National Screening Committee standards. The use of a low frequency probe will facilitate better penetration and improved views but the operator will also need to consider placement of probe. Scanning below the apron of fat and over the umbilicus, the two thinner parts of the abdominal wall may aid ultrasound visualisation. In addition, a combination

Figure 3.1. First trimester scan in a woman with an increased BMI. Left pre-optimisation Right post – optimisation

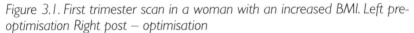

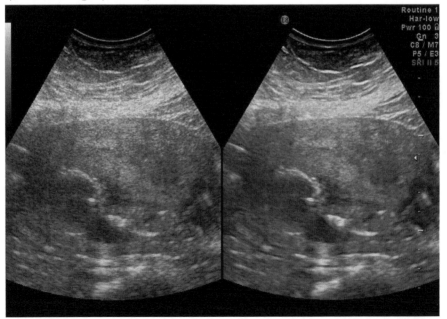

of transabdominal and transvaginal ultrasound examination may be needed to optimise views. Transvaginal scanning improves views of the fetal structures particularly in the first trimester and may be preferable to the operator. However, a transvaginal approach is more invasive for the woman than a transabdominal approach. Therefore having a lower threshold for the use of this may be less acceptable to women.

As well as being technically demanding, ultrasound examinations of obese women is also more physically challenging for the operator. The incidence of musculo-skeletal pain and discomfort among sonographers is approximately 80% (Gregrory 1999). When scanning an obese patient the operator needs to grip the transducer and apply sustained pressure with a flexed or hyperextended wrist to obtain adequate views. In addition to this, there is often an increased scan time to complete the examination. All of these factors increase the risk of RSI among this group of health care professionals. Managers of ultrasound screening units should ensure that staff are aware of methods to prevent RSI. Provision should also be made to ensure staff are aware of the maximum loads for scanning couches and bariatric couches are available when required.

Subfertility and miscarriage

There is a higher prevalence of irregular menstrual cycles, amenorrhoea and subfertility among obese women. This is likely to be due to the increased occurrence of polycystic ovarian syndrome (PCOS); approximately 35-40% of all women with PCOS are obese (Franks 1989). In addition, obesity is associated with an increased risk of first trimester loss and recurrent miscarriage; the risk of miscarriage before the first live born child is 25-37% higher in obese women (Hamilton-Fairley et al 1992). This is among both women with PCOS and those with normal ovarian morphology. The underlying cause of this is not completely understood, although it has been suggested that the risk of spontaneous miscarriage rises as insulin resistance increases. Metformin, an insulin sensitising agent, has been found to reduce miscarriage rates, which is in keeping with this hypothesis (Glueck et al 2004).

Fertility treatment for obese women is also complex. Obesity is believed to have a negative impact on subfertility treatment and if conception occurs there is an increased risk of pregnancy loss. With ovulation induction, obese women are up to three times more likely to miscarry, and with egg donation and IVF this increases to four times more likely (Fedorcsak et al 2000).

Ultrasound therefore has a particularly important role to play in confirming the viability of a pregnancy, accurately dating the pregnancy, and diagnosing multiple pregnancy. The accuracy of pregnancy dating ultrasounds however can be decreased in obese women when using transabdominal scanning. This is because of reduced image clarity and therefore transvaginal scanning is often recommended.

Congenital abnormalities

Maternal obesity, independent of diabetes, is associated with a range of structural anomalies. Congenital structural anomalies are a leading cause of stillbirth, infant mortality, and are also important contributors to preterm birth and childhood morbidity. There is a broad spectrum of malformations that are associated with maternal obesity (Stothard et al 2009) *(Table 3.1)*.

The mechanisms that link obesity and congenital anomalies are not fully understood and several hypotheses have been suggested. Maternal obesity has been associated with nutritional deficiencies, specifically reduced folate levels (Anderson 2005). Several studies (Anderson 2005; Martinez-Frias

Table 3.1. Demonstrates congenital anomalies which have been associated with obesity.

Congenital anomalies associated with obesity	Congenital anomalies not associated with obesity
Neural Tube Defects • Anencephaly • Spina Bifida	• Encephalocele
Cardiovascular Anomalies • Septal Anomalies	Cardiovascular Anomalies • Tetralogy of Fallot • Transposition of the great arteries
Orofacial Clefts • Cleft palate • Cleft lip and palate	Orofacial Clefts • Cleft lip
Other Congenital Anomalies • Anorectal atresia • Hydrocephaly • Limb reduction anomaly	Other Congenital Anomalies • Gastroschisis • Diaphragmatic hernia • Oesophageal atresia • Hypospadias • microcephaly • microtia/anotia

2005) have found a two fold increase in the risk for spina bifida among obese mothers compared with mothers of recommended BMI. It has been suggested that the protective effect of folic acid in reducing the risk of a neural tube defect may not be observed in obese women (Werler et al 1996). A case control surveillance programme found that a daily intake of 400 mcg was protective against neural tube defects in infants of women weighing less than 70 kg but not in infants of women weighing more than 70 kg (Werler at al 1996). It may therefore be beneficial to consider offering this group of women a high dose (5 mg) folic acid supplement. It is also intriguing to note that many of the congenital anomalies listed above have similar developmental timing and responsiveness to folic acid which suggests a possible common underlying aetiology. Deficiencies in other nutrients may also underlie the association with other congenital anomalies.

Furthermore, obesity and diabetes share similar metabolic abnormalities, including insulin resistance and hyperglycaemia. Obesity is a strong risk factor for type 2 diabetes and maternal diabetes is an established risk factor for congenital anomalies, particularly neural tube defects and cardiac malformations (Martinez-Frias et al 2005). Therefore undiagnosed diabetes and hyperglycaemia in obese pregnant women is one potential explanation for the increased risk of congenital anomalies. It is possible that prepregnancy diagnosis of diabetes may permit intervention prior to conception and that obese women planning a pregnancy should be screened for diabetes and treated if appropriate. It could therefore be proposed that weight reduction and good glycaemic control could help reduce the rates of congenital abnormality in this high risk group.

Prenatal diagnosis of congenital malformations

The National Screening Committee recommend that all women in the UK are offered two routine ultrasound examinations in pregnancy to screen for structural malformations, the first at 11 to 13+6 weeks and the second, a detailed anomaly scan at 18 to 20+6 weeks gestation. The purpose of the scan at 11 to 13+6 weeks is to confirm viability, accurately date the pregnancy, diagnose multiple pregnancy, screen for major structural malformations and to offer screening for Down's Syndrome. Continuously improving ultrasound equipment and a better understanding of fetal development have fuelled the quest for earlier prenatal diagnosis and interventions, and this is now possible for some congenital abnormalities. For example, the diagnosis of acrania (absent cranial vault – *Figure 3.2*) or an anterior abdominal wall defect (exomphalos – *Figure 3.3*) should be routinely made at this scan. However in obese women, the distance between the probe and fetus at this

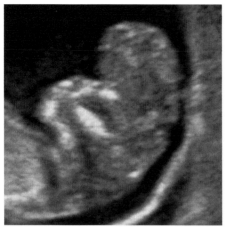

Figure 3.2. Acrania diagnosed in the first trimester

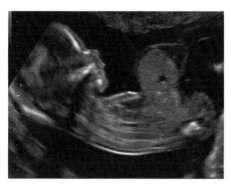

Figure 3.3. Abdominal wall defect - exomphalos

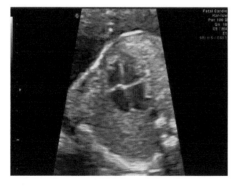

Figure 3.4. Four chamber view of the heart

early gestation makes visualisation of the major structures extremely difficult and it may be necessary to use transvaginal ultrasound. Transvaginal ultrasound is limited by having reduced manoeuvrability and in some cases this may prevent complete examination. This may include measurement of nuchal translucency thickness at this gestation which can reduce the detection of anueploidy in these women.

The purpose of the 18 to 20+6 week scan is to provide information for women so that they are able to exercise informed choice. The aim is to identify abnormalities either incompatible with life, or associated with morbidity and abnormalities that may benefit from antenatal or postnatal intervention. However, the reduced ability to visualise fetal structures, particularly cardiac (*Figure 3.4*) and craniospinal (*Figure 3.5*), in obese women has a significant impact on the detection rate of structural anomalies. Wong et al (2002) reported that the detection rate for structural anomalies in obese women was 30% compared to 73% in the diabetic non obese women. It is therefore important that health care professionals are aware that even with heightened surveillance ultrasound, practitioners are more likely to miss structural abnormalities in this high risk group. Health care professionals counselling obese women need to inform parents that the detection rate for structural malformations may be lower.

In addition, women's expectations of pregnancy ultrasound may be greater than what is realistically achievable, for example, obtaining a clear image of the baby's face for the parents to take away. It is advisable to forewarn parents that this may not always be possible in order to manage expectations.

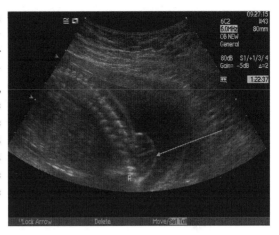

Figure 3.5. Spina Bifida in a 20 week fetus

Invasive testing/fetal therapy

In cases where there is an increased risk of a chromosomal abnormality, such as first trimester combined screening for Down's Syndrome, parents are offered invasive prenatal diagnosis. Invasive procedures such as amniocentesis and chorionic villus sampling (CVS) involve insertion of fine needle into the uterus to obtain tissue from the pregnancy which can be examined in the laboratory. These procedures carry a small risk (1-2%) of miscarriage due to the invasive nature of the test. Fetal therapies also utilise the same approach and therefore carry a small risk of miscarriage, these include intrauterine transfusion for fetal anaemia and laser ablation for Twin to Twin Transfusion Syndrome (TTTS).

All invasive procedures require continuous ultrasound monitoring in order to minimise the risk of miscarriage and inadvertent fetal harm (*Figure 3.6*). Visualisation of the needle through the sub-cutaneous abdominal fat worsens with increasing thickness and density. This is exaggerated by the fact that the needles may not be long enough to reach the desired target. In this situation needles which

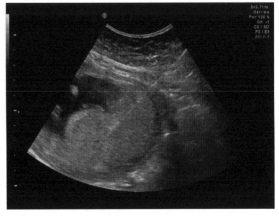

Figure 3.6 Ultrasound guided Chorionic Villus Sampling

have a wider gauge and are longer in length may have to be used. However the length increases the flexibility of the needle, making a controlled approach more difficult. Overall these factors are likely to increase the risk of miscarriage from invasive prenatal diagnosis or therapy.

Hypertensive disorders in pregnancy and disorders of fetal growth

Hypertension, pre eclampsia (PE), intrauterine growth restriction and macrosomia are all known risk factors for perinatal morbidity and mortality. Independent of pregnancy, the association between hypertension and adiposity is well documented. Elevated BMI is an independent risk factor for the development of pregnancy induced hypertension (Erez-Weiss et al 2005). Even when the degree of excess body mass is moderate, the incidence of hypertension and PE is significantly higher in comparison with control patients (O'Brien et al 2003). A systematic review of maternal BMI and risk of PE showed that the risk of PE is typically doubled with each 5 to 7 kg/m2 increase in prepregnancy BMI. In addition to this, PE is associated with a significantly increased risk of intrauterine growth restriction. Conversely, there is a two fold increase in the risk of macrosomia among obese women (Hall and Neubert 2005). The risks of macrosomia are well documented and include antepartum stillbirth, prolonged labour, operative delivery, emergency section, post partum haemorragh (PPH), shoulder dystocia and perineal trauma.

Routine antenatal care guidance recommends palpation of the maternal abdomen and measurement of the symphyseal fundal height to screen for disorders of fetal growth. In obese women this is often not useful and ultrasound may have a role to play in routinely assessing fetal growth in the third trimester. Evidence is lacking on the optimum timing and frequency of scans in these women but it may be beneficial to perform ultrasound examinations at 28 and 36 weeks gestation. This enables the operator to estimate the fetal weight at term and confirm the presentation which may be difficult to ascertain on abdominal palpation. It is important to note that the accuracy of sonographic birth weight prediction is adversely affected by obesity.

A combination of ultrasound and maternal serum biochemistry can be utilised to screen for PE and intrauterine growth restriction. Abnormal uterine artery Doppler waveforms *(Figure 3.7 and 3.8)* and low levels (<0.25 multiples of the median (MoM's) of pregnancy associated plasma protein – A (PAPP-A) are useful in predicting PE and intrauterine growth restriction from as early as the first trimester (Pilalis et al 2007).

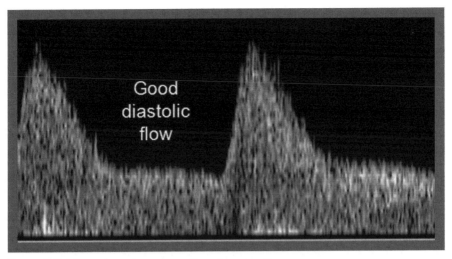

Figure 3.7. Normal uterine artery Doppler waveform

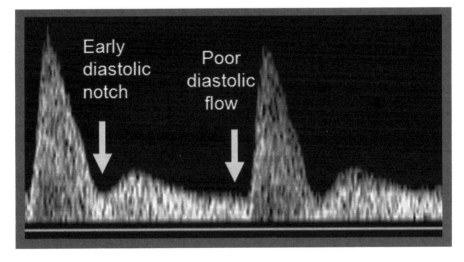

Figure 3.8. Abnormal uterine artery Doppler waveform

Stillbirth

Several studies have suggested that obesity is associated with an increased risk of antepartum stillbirth (Cedergren 2004; Cnattingius 1998). This may, in part, be due to the increased prevalence of congenital malformation and diabetes in this cohort of women. However when excluding for these risk factors, the overall risk is still increased and therefore there are additional factors which at present are unknown.

Ultrasound has a role in the detection of structural malformations and aberrant fetal growth, however it is unable to accurately predict those pregnancies at risk of still birth where the fetus appears to be normally grown and structurally normal. Unfortunately management strategies to prevent stillbirth have not been rigorously studied in this population. The use of kick charts is a reasonable and low cost technique but has not been evaluated in a randomised trial.

Prolonged pregnancy

The higher a woman's prepregnancy BMI, the more likely she is to have a post dates pregnancy (Stotland et al 2007) which is associated with induction of labour, increased risk of operative delivery as well as neonatal morbidity and mortality. It has been suggested that serial membrane sweeping from 38 weeks gestation may reduce the risk of the pregnancy continuing beyond 41 weeks gestation, however this gives no indication of placental function or fetal wellbeing in those pregnancy's that continue beyond 41 weeks.

Ultrasound assessment of fetal wellbeing and measurement of cervical length at 40-41 weeks gestation can also assess placental function, identify previously undiagnosed problems that may benefit from an elective caesarean section and predict the chances of spontaneous labour in the next 7-10 days. This type of examination has been shown to reduce induction of labour rates and may be of benefit to inform management of prolonged pregnancy in this cohort of women (Rao et al 2008).

In summary, ultrasound has a very important role to play in the management of obese women. However sub-optimal views reduce the detection rate of structural malformation, decrease the accuracy of fetal weight estimation, and complicate invasive procedures. It is therefore important that health professional's ensure women with an increased BMI are counselled fully about the both the benefits and limitations of obstetric ultrasound.

References

Department of Health (2003) Health Survey for England 2002 – Latest Trends. http://www.dh.gov.uk/en/publicationsandstatistics/publishedsurvey/healthsurveyforengland/healthsurveyresults/ (accessed 3rd March 2009).

Anderson JL, Waller DK, Canfield MA *et al* (2005) Maternal obesity, gestational diabetes and central nervous system birth defects. *Epidemiology* **16**: 87–92

Cedergren MI (2004) Maternal morbid obesity and the risk of adverse pregnancy outcome.

Obstetrics & Gynaecology **103**: 219–24

Cnattingius S, Bergstrom R, Lipworth L *et al* (1998) Prepregnancy weight and the risk of adverse pregnancy outcomes. *New England Journal of Medicine* **338**: 147–52

Erez-Weiss I, Erez O, Shoham-Vardi I *et al* (2005) The association between maternal obesity, glucose intolerance and hypertensive disorders of pregnancy in non-diabetic pregnant women. *Hypertens pregnancy* **24**: 125–36

Fedorcsak P, Storeng R, Dale PO *et al* (2000) Obesity is a risk factor for early pregnancy loss after IVF or ICSI. *Acta Obstet Gynecol Scand* **79**: 43–8

Franks S (1989) Polycystic ovary syndrome: a changing perspective. *Clinical Endocrinology* **31**: 87–120

Glueck CJ, Wang P, Goldenberg N *et al* (2004) Pregnancy loss, polycystic ovary syndrome, thrombophilia, hypofibrinolysis, enoxaparin, metformin. *Clin Appl Thromb Hemost* **10**: 323–324

Gregrory V (1999) Occupational Health and Safety update: Report on the results of an Australian Sonography Survey on prevalence of musculoskeletal disorders among Sonographers.

http://www.a-s-a.com.au/p_ohs/documents/OH&S%20update%2Dec.99pdf (accessed 3rd March 2009).

Hall LF, Nuebert AG (2005) Obesity and Pregnancy. *Obstetrical and Gynecological Survey* **60**(4): 253–60

Hamilton-Fairley D, Kiddy D, Watson H *et al* (1992) Association of moderate obesity with poor pregnancy outcome in women with polycystic ovary syndrome treated with low dose gonadotrophin. *British Journal of Obstetrics & Gynaecology* **99**:128–31

Martinez-Friars ML, Friars JP, Bermejo E (2005) Pre-gestational body mass index predicts an increased risk of congenital malformations in infants of mothers with gestational diabetes. *Diabet Med* **22**: 775–81

O'Brien TE, Ray JG, Chan WS (2003) Maternal body mass index and the risk of pre-eclampsia: a systematic overview. *Epidemiology* **14**: 368–74

Pilalis A, Souka AP, Antsaklis P *et al* (2007) Screening for pre-eclampsia and fetal growth restriction by uterine artery Doppler and PAPP-A at 11–14 weeks' gestation. *Ultrasound Obstet Gynecol* **29**:135–40

Rao A, Celik E, Poggi S *et al* (2008) Cervical Length and Maternal Factors in expectantly managed prolonged pregnancy: prediction of onset of labour and mode of delivery. *Ultrasound in Obstetrics & Gynaecology* **32**: 646–51

Stotland NE, Washington AE, Caughey AB (2007) Prepregnancy body mass index and length of gestation at term. *American Journal of Obstetrics and Gynecology* **197**: 378

Stothard KJ, Tennant PWG, Bell R *et al* (2009) Maternal Overweight and Obesity and the Risk of Congenital Anomalies. A Systematic Review and Meta-analysis. *JAMA* **301**(6): 636–50

Werler MM, Louik C, Shapiro S *et al* (1996) Prepregnant weight in relation to the risks of neural tube defects. *JAMA* **275**: 1089–92

Wolfe HM, Sokol TJ, Martier SM *et al* (1990) Maternal obesity: a potential source of error in sonographic prenatal diagnosis. *Obstetrics & Gynaecology* **76**: 339–42

Wong SF, Chan FY, Cincotta RB *et al* (2002) Routine ultrasound screening in diabetic pregnancies. *Ultrasound in Obstetrics & Gynaecology* **19**: 171–6

Chapter 4

Antenatal Assessment and Care

Yana Richens and Tina Lavender

Introduction

The headlines in the newspapers, "Obesity is biggest threat to women during pregnancy" (Hope 2007), following the latest publication of the Saving Mothers Lives (Confidential Enquiry into Maternal and Child Health CEMACH 2007a) were of no surprise to most midwives. Midwives have been aware of, and dealing with, the problems associated with obesity during pregnancy for several years; so what has changed? Why are we so concerned with obesity now? The fact is that the current obesity epidemic in the general population has brought the problem to the attention of the government, the health service, the media and the public. Unsurprisingly, therefore, an increasing number of women who are classified as obese are becoming pregnant.

The problem is so serious that the government has published national guidance on the care and management of the obese adult; however this does not extend to pregnant women (DH 2007a). The guidance is a stepped approach and could be easily utilised in midwifery practice along with the guidance on "Raising the Issue of weight with adults" (DH 2007b).

This chapter aims to provide midwives with guidance on the management of women with a raised BMI in the antentatal period, based on current best evidence and the authors experience of managing a clinic for women with raised BMI.

As we have already read earlier in the book, the Body Mass Index (BMI) is the most commonly used measure to classify obesity. The BMI uses weight in relation to height and is defined as weight in kilograms divided by the square of height in square metres. Adults with a BMI ≥ 30 are classified as obese. *Table 4.1* shows the classification used by the Institute of Medicine, World Health Organisation and National Institute of Health and Clinical Excellence.

Table 4.1 Classification of obesity	
Classification	**BMI (kg/m²)**
Normal Range	18.5-24.9
Overweight	25.0 -29.9
Obese Class I	30.0 -34.9
Obese Class II	35.0 -39.9
Obese Class III (Morbid obesity)	≥ 40

Early antenatal assessment (booking)

It is essential that when a midwife undertakes an antenatal booking that this is used as part of the overall clinical assessment of the woman, in order to plan the optimal care for her during the pregnancy. The reason why this is so important is that it enables a safe co-ordinated approach to care to women who are obese during pregnancy. A full risk assessment and forward planning for this group of women is pivotal to a safe pregnancy and positive outcomes. It is important that all women are given respect and treated as an individual, as highlighted in CEMACH (2007a):

> "*Of the two morbidly obese women who died in their first trimester, one actively avoided doctors and midwives completely. Morbid obesity is a distressing condition and sufferers may find it difficult to talk to clinicians for fear of stigmatisation.*" (CEMACH 2007a:56)

Women should be made aware of the risks of having a raised BMI. They should also be made aware of the planned management strategies to minimise these risks; these may include thromboprophylaxis regimes, place of birth, mode of birth, and dietary advice. All aspects of management of care during the antenatal, intrapartum and postnatal period, should be discussed with the woman and clearly documented in the maternity hand held records notes; this must be in partnership with the woman.

The reason why recognition of obesity associated complications are so important was first highlighted within the CEMACH "Why Mothers Die 2000-2002" (2004) report; 78 women who died from direct or indirect causes (35% of maternal deaths in these categories) were obese with a BMI of 30 or more and of these over 20% had a BMI 35 or greater. The latest CEMACH report (2007) reported that out of the 295 women who died from causes directly or indirectly related to pregnancy during the period of 2003-2005, over half were overweight or obese. It should also be recognized that a BMI itself may not be the direct cause for a maternal death, as there are likely to be a number of causative associated factors including specific health problems and social deprivation. As health care professionals we are aware of and often deal with these problems. Women themselves, however, are not always aware of these significant health risks to themselves or their baby during pregnancy. Both midwives and health care professional have a duty of care to inform women of these potential problems.

Maternal and fetal risks

It is recognised that maternal and fetal risks increase as BMI rises. This has been highlighted throughout the earlier chapters in the book. Pregnant women with a BMI ≥30 have a significantly increased risk of thromboembolism, hypertension, cardiac problems, pre eclampsia (PE), and gestational diabetes (Sebire et al 2001; Weiss et al 2004). These women also have an increased risk of anaesthetic complications, sleep apnoea, postpartum haemorrhage and fetal risks e.g. stillbirth, neonatal death and shoulder dystocia (Cedergren 2004; Usha Kiran 2005). There is also a much higher Caesarean section (CS) rate in this group of women (Chu 2007). *Table 4.2* highlights some of the complications associated with obesity in pregnancy, which have been documented in the published literature.

The question is: how should we support this group of women? Some hospitals have implemented specific clinics for this group of women; the impact of these clinics on morbidity and mortality is currently unknown. However, at least the women attending these clinics receive focused information and support.

Table 4.2 Obesity related complications

• Infertility	• Slow labours
• Miscarriage	• Fetal macrosomia
• Fetal birth defects, especially neural tube defect	• Thrombo-phlebitis
• Implantation disorders	• Thromboembolism
• Urinary tract infection	• Post Caesarean and wound infection
• Gestational diabetes	• Post-partum haemorrhage
• Type 2 diabetes	• Stillbirth and neonatal death
• Hypertension, pre eclampsia and eclampsia	• Maternal death

The introduction of a Maternal Nutrition Clinic at University College London Hospital (UCLH)

The antenatal clinic at UCLH was started in response to the findings of the CEMACH (2004). Initially there was skepticism amongst health professionals over "another specialist clinic', however the barriers to implementation were overcome due to the support of midwives, obstetricians and managers, and the clear clinical need.

One of the dilemmas when starting such a clinic is what it should be called. The clinic at UCLH was named a Maternal Nutrition Clinic' as it was believed to be less offensive to women. Others have chosen 'Obesity clinic' or 'Bariatric clinic'; to date there is no information about how women feel about these names.

The clinic is now led and managed by one of the authors (Yana Richens). The clinic is specifically aimed at women with a BMI ≥35. It is anticipated that this will be phased out in the near future with all health professionals who are providing maternity care being responsible for safe and appropriate management of these women.

The purpose of the clinic is to provide the women with one-to-one care, with a focus on weight management and healthy eating during pregnancy. Its objectives are:

- To offer a partnership in care, to provide women with the optimum opportunity for good maternal and fetal outcomes.
- Maintenance of dignity and self-esteem for the woman.
- Ensuring that processes are in place to maximise the safety of mother and baby during pregnancy, labour and delivery.
- Support to other midwives providing care.
- To monitor appropriate pregnancy outcomes.

The clinic is held at the hospital due to centralization of equipment. Midwives working in a community setting will not always have access to the correct equipment required for this group of women. The clinic has bariatric sit on scales so that women can be weighed accurately. A further reason for this clinic being located in the hospital is due to the fact that in central London a large percentage of women wishing to have their baby at the hospital do not live in the locality.

Both midwives and doctors can refer directly to the clinic and an appointment is made centrally by booking an appointment with the receptionist in the antenatal clinic. A copy of the care plan is available in the woman's medical notes. This first visit is not intended to be an extra visit but is part of the woman's normal antenatal care

For women with a BMI of ≥35, referral to a consultant obstetrician is made at:

- 22 weeks for consideration of the management plan for pregnancy. At the same time an appointment to see the consultant anaesthetist is made.
- 36 weeks following ultra sound scan for size/growth and presentation of the fetus, to discuss plan for labour and birth.

Due to the increase in the number of women with a BMI over 30 the clinic has designed two care pathways, one for women with a BMI of 30–34.9 and one for women with a BMI ≥35. These will be discussed in detail later. The woman should have one dedicated midwife responsible for coordinating her care. This midwife will offer support and advocacy, guiding her through the variety of additional services that may be required.

> The assessment of risk should be made with the pregnant woman every time she makes contact with a health professional during her pregnancy.

Booking visit

The assessment of a pregnant woman's BMI should be made at the booking appointment, ideally less than 12 weeks gestation (NICE 2008; CEMACH 2007).

All women must be commenced on folic acid 5mg daily, ideally before pregnancy, or, if this has not occurred, as soon as pregnancy is confirmed, up to 12 weeks' gestation. Studies have linked maternal obesity with an increased risk of neural tube defects, however the mechanism for this is not clearly understood (Watkins et al 2003; Cedergren et al 2004; Waller et al 2007). It is proposed that obese women require higher levels of folate. A large case-control study found that a daily intake of at least 400 mg of folic acid reduced the risk of neural tube defect-affected pregnancy by 40% in women weighing 70 kg, with no risk reduction observed in women weighing more than 70 kg (Werler et al 1996). It is interesting to note that in Scotland, for the first time, a sharp rise in the increase of babies born with spina bifida (RCM 2009) has been observed. In 2007 the Scottish Public Health Observatory published a report which highlighted that only America has a higher percentage of overweight adults than in Scotland (Grant et al 2007). Although obesity among Scottish and English men are broadly the same, Scottish women are more likely to be obese than women in England.

All women should have their height and weight measured by the health professional carrying out the booking visit, rather than using self-reported measurements. Height, weight and calculated BMI should be recorded. If there are no scales available in the community, for example when home booking, this should be clearly documented and the woman weighed at the earliest opportunity. Women should be weighed at every antenatal visit, and this should be recorded in the woman's hand held notes. The NICE Antenatal Care Guideline (2008) recommends that repeated weight measurements during pregnancy should occur only in circumstances where clinical management is likely to be influenced. However, it is worth remembering when recording a BMI that this measurement does not account for body fat distribution. More recently, it has been recommended that the treatment of obesity need to focus more on abdominal fat and not BMI (Despres et al 2001). The ethnicity of the individual also needs to be considered as individuals from a south Asians background are considered overweight when BMI greater than 23 kg/m^2.

Women with a BMI ≥30 have a higher risk of complications during labour including dysfunctional labour and postpartum haemorrhage. Fetal heart rate monitoring is also more technically difficult. For these reasons women with a BMI ≥30 should be advised to labour and give birth on the consultant obstetric-led unit.

A history should be taken of any significant pre-existing and past medical conditions e.g. diabetes, raised blood pressure, cardiac problems and sleep apnoea, any personal history of deep vein thrombosis, pulmonary embolism and known thrombophilia. Referrals should be made as appropriate for follow up of any medical conditions identified. It is known that nearly half of the 31 women with a known BMI who died of a thromboembolic event were obese (CEMACH 2007). All women should be assessed and a referral should be made to the haematologist for assessment if there is personal or family history of deep vein thrombosis or pulmonary embolism. The importance of mobility is also discussed with the woman.

It is essential that correct weight adjusted doses of prophylactic and therapeutic doses of low molecular weight heparin are prescribed to women. The importance of this was highlighted in the case of the woman who was prescribed the correct prophylactic dose of tinzaparin for a 90kg woman however she weighted 200kg and sadly died (CEMACH 2007). Care was judged to be sub-standard in two thirds (22 of the 33) of cases of pulmonary embolism in the CEMACH report. The main reason given for this was inadequate risk assessment in early pregnancy. As there are no current national guidelines for screening of risk factors for venous thromboembolism in pregnancy, *Table 4.3* summarises the Royal College of Obstetricians guideline (RCOG 2004) for thromboprophylaxis in pregnancy, this provides an excellent antentatal check list.

In line with the NICE antenatatal care guideline (2008) this group of

Table 4.3 Royal College of Obstetricians and Gynaecologists (RCOG 2004) guidelines for thromboprophylaxis in pregnancy, labour and after vaginal delivery and CS

Risk factors for venous thromboembolism in pregnancy and the puerperium (a)

Pre-existing	New onset or transient (b)
Previous VTE	Surgical procedure in pregnancy or puerperium, e.g. evacuation of retained products of conception, postpartum sterilisation
Thrombophilia	
congenital	
antithrombin deficiency	
protein C deficiency	
protein S deficiency	Hyperemesis
Factor V Leiden	Dehydration
prothrombin gene variant	Ovarian hyperstimulation
acquired (antiphospholipid	syndrome
syndrome)	Severe infection, e.g. pyelonephritis
lupus anticoagulant	Immobility (> 4 days bed rest)
anticardiolipin antibodies	Pre eclampsia
Age over 35 years	Excessive blood loss
Obesity (BMI > 30 kg/m2)	Long-haul travel
either prepregnancy	
or in early pregnancy	Prolonged labour (c)
Parity > 4	Midcavity instrumental delivery (c)
Gross varicose veins	Immobility after delivery (c)
Paraplegia	
Sickle cell disease	
Inflammatory disorders e.g.	
inflammatory bowel disease	
Some medical disorders, e.g.	
nephrotic syndrome,	
certain cardiac diseases	
Myeloproliferative disorders,	
e.g. essential thrombocythaemia,	
polycythaemia vera	

(a) Although these are all accepted as thromboembolic risk factors, there are few data to support the degree of increased risk associated with many of them
(b) These risk factors are potentially reversible and may develop at later stages in gestation than the initial risk assessment or may resolve; an ongoing individual risk assessment is important
(c) Risk factors specific to postpartum VTE only

women require screening for diabetes see box below for recommendations on screening for gestational diabetes. As highlighted on the care pathway this is not a one off investigation, and a Random Blood sugar will be taken again at 28 weeks. For women with a BMI over 35 a glucose tolerance test is routinely undertaken.

Recommendations on screening for gestational diabetes

Screening for gestational diabetes using risk factors is recommended in a healthy population. At the booking appointment, the following risk factors for gestational diabetes should be determined:

- BMI above 30 kg/mg
- Previous macrosomic baby weighing 4.5 kg or above
- Previous gestational diabetes (refer to 'Diabetes in pregnancy' (NICE 2008) Clinical Guideline 63
- Family history of diabetes (first-degree relative with diabetes)
- Family origin with a high prevalence of diabetes.

South Asian (specifically women whose country of family origin is India, Pakistan or Bangladesh) black Caribbean Middle Eastern (specifically women whose country of family origin is Saudi Arabia, United Arab Emirates, Iraq, Jordan, Syria, Oman, Qatar, Kuwait, Lebanon or Egypt). Women with any one of these risk factors should be offered testing for gestational diabetes (refer to'Diabetes in pregnancy' [NICE 2008 Clinical Guideline 63).

Antenatal care

Women with a BMI ≥30 are at higher risk of complications during pregnancy and due to this the number of antenatal visits reflect the risk. As proposed by NICE (2008):

A schedule of antenatal appointments should be determined by the function of the appointments. (NICE 2008:72).

Currently we have two care pathways which reflect this (*Table 4.4*). *Figure 4.1* is for women with a BMI of 30–34.9, and *Figure 4.2* for women with a BMI over 35, there are 10 recommended visits for this group of women regardless of parity. Women with a BMI greater than 35 often request an antenatal check at 40 weeks.

Table 4.4 Care pathways for obese women	
Obese Class I **BMI 30–34.9**	**Obese Class II** **BMI 35.0 –**
Midwife to book and risk assess refer appropriately	Midwife to book and risk assess refer appropriately
Suitable for shared community care Consultant Midwife 16 wks Consultant Obstetrician 36weeks / earlier if required Anaesthetist 22 weeks	Consultant care Consultant Midwife 16 wks Consultant Obstetrician 22 weeks Anaesthetist 22 weeks
Advice re healthy diet. Refer to dietician via GP if target weight gain exceeded during pregnancy.	Advice re healthy diet. Referral to dietician via GP at booking
Scans 12 week 20 week detailed anomaly scan 36 week scan if needed	Scans 12 week 20 week detailed anomaly scan Scan 36 weeks presentation position and size prior to delivery plan
GTT at 28 weeks. Refer to diabetic team if required	GTT at 12 weeks GTT at 28 weeks Refer to diabetic team if required
Blood pressure and urinalysis should be assessed as per the antenatal guideline. Remember increased risk of pre-eclampsia -observe as appropriate	Blood pressure and urinalysis should be assessed From 24- 32 weeks-3 weekly After 32 weeks –every 2 weeks – if symptomatic follow hypertension guideline
	Hospital review 36-37 weeks gestation by senior obstetrician regarding mode of delivery

Weight gain during pregnancy

It has been suggested that pregnancy is not a time to lose weight; this advice is reinforced by families and the lay media. However the antenatal booking is an ideal time to provide women with health promotional messages. Women who have been identified as obese/morbidly obese should be encouraged to discuss their diet and the effects that obesity can cause during pregnancy, in much the same way that smoking is discussed. Recent studies suggest that providing an intervention programme to support women to lose weight during pregnancy may be beneficial, leading to postpartum weight loss, despite not effecting delivery or neonatal outcome (Claesson et al

BMI's 30 –34.9

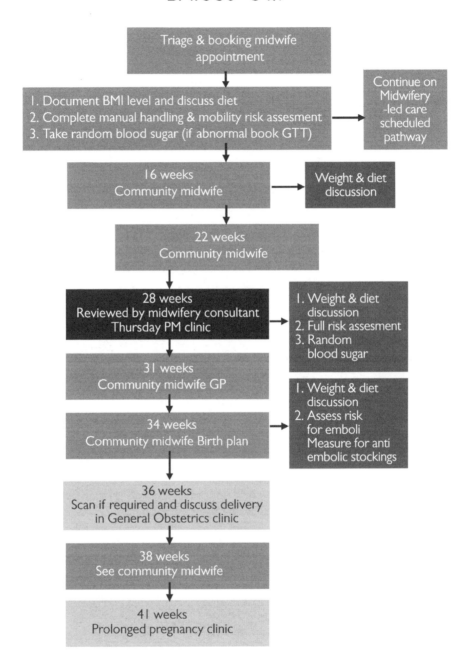

Figure 4.1 Pathway for women with a BMI 30 – 34.9

BMI ≥35

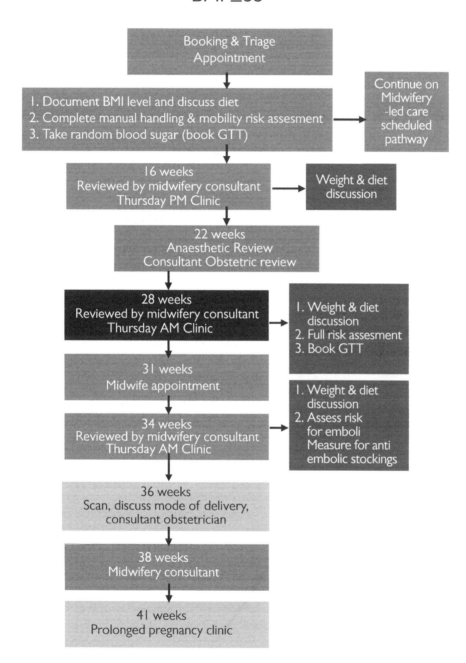

Figure 4.2 Pathway for women with BMI over 35

2007; O'Toole et al 2003; Jevitt 2005). Olafsdottir et al (2006) identified that women with a BMI of 25-29.9 kg/m2 before pregnancy were most likely to gain excessive weight, and be categorised as obese after pregnancy. This could significantly lead to complications in any further pregnancy as Villamor & Cnattingius (2006) identified that a weight gain of 3 BMI units after pregnancy was significantly associated with the risk of stillbirth deliveries in subsequent pregnancies. *Table 4.5* provides a guide to weight gain during pregnancy (Institutue of Medicine 2009). Atlhough dieting is not recommended if women eat the required calorific intake as proposed in Chapter 5 they will lose weight without adverse outcomes. It is important to be aware that some women who are overweight also experience elements of social exclusion and low self esteem e.g. unemployment and low income (CEMACH 2007), therefore any dietary advice should take into account the woman's circumstances.

Table 4.5 Weight gain recommended in pregnancy for different BMI categories Institute of Medicine (2009)			
Weight category	BMI	Recommended weight gain in Kg during pregnancy	Mean Kg / week
Underweight	<18.5	12.5 – 18.0kg	0.5
Normal weight	18.5 – 24.9	11.5 – 16.0 kg	0.4
Overweight	25 - 29.9	7.0 – 11.5 kg	0.3
Obese	>30	5.0 – 9.0kg	0.2

Abdominal palpation

As midwives we need to be more sensitive to the body image of this group of women and caution needs to be observed in both verbal and non verbal communications. Women should not be allowed to self denigrate; any negative comments or half hearted comments should be met with a positive response. This group of women is very aware of how society perceives them and it maybe the first time for many of them that they have exposed their bodies to anyone other than their partner. Prior to undertaking an abdominal palpation it is sometimes an idea to warn the woman that you may not be able to hear the fetal heart beat straight away, if at all, with the sonicaid and this is due to the adipose tissue. However you may find that if the woman helps by lifting the apron of fat, the fetal heart can be heard. It may also be that at this examination you find the woman has a thrush infection in her groins, as she is unable to wash and dry these areas as the pregnancy increases; she will require practical advice on how to manage this for example to use a shower chair and sit and lift the apron of fat and wash and dry throughly.. Fundal height measurements may not be a reliable means of estimating fetal growth. For this reason, exta ultrasound scans maybe requred at 28 and 36 weeks. A scan at 36 weeks is useful for presentation, fetal growth and estimated fetal weight.

If the woman perceives any reduction in fetal movement after 28 weeks, or a change in movement patterns, she must be advised to contact the maternity unit; often morbidly obese women experience difficulty in identifying fetal movements, a factor that needs to be discussed with her.

Blood pressure

In accordance with the NICE guideline (2007), a blood pressure measurement and urinalysis for protein should be carried out at each antenatal visit to screen for PE.

More frequent blood pressure measurements should be considered for pregnant women who have a BMI over 30. Very clear guidelines on how to take the woman's blood pressure are provided by NICE (2008)

Blood pressure should be measured as outlined below:

- Remove tight clothing, ensure arm is relaxed and supported at heart level
- Use cuff of appropriate size
- Inflate cuff to 20–30 mmHg above palpated systolic blood pressure
- Lower column slowly, by 2 mmHg per second or per beat
- Read blood pressure to the nearest 2 mmHg
- Measure diastolic blood pressure as disappearance of sounds (phase V).

Hypertension, in which there is a single diastolic blood pressure of 110 mmHg or two consecutive readings of 90 mmHg at least 4 hours apart and/or significant proteinuria (1+), should prompt increased surveillance.

If the systolic blood pressure is above 160 mmHg on two consecutive readings at least 4 hours apart, treatment should be considered (NICE 2007).

When monitoring blood pressure, an appropriate size cuff must be used. If automated systems are used to monitor blood pressure it is important to ensure that these have been validated for use in pregnancy as some underestimate systolic pressure in PE. The Action on Pre-Eclampsia web site also has further guidelines and information on equipment (APEC 2010).

Overleaf is a summary of the main points to remember during the antentatal period.

Antenatal Check list for women with a BMI over 30:

- Book women as early as possible for consultant care where possible continuity of care by the same midwife.
- Pre-existing medical problems to have appropriate and timely referral
- Discuss weight openly (women are aware that they are obese), provide advice on healthy eating and suggest a food diary so that you can read this at the next antenatal visit. Identify how much help and support the woman has to lose weight sensibly and refer to a dietician if help is required.
- Women with severe obesity (BMI greater than 35 kg/m^2) plus one additional risk factor for hypertensive disease should be prescribed aspirin 75 mg/day from 12 weeks.
- Folic acid 5mg per day.
- Discuss problems associated with obesity and pregnancy to both the woman and the baby.
- Schedule of antenatal care to reflect risk. Use ultrasound to detect Fetal Heart when necessary, and give fetal movement chart from 28 weeks gestation (this is due to the fact that some women do not feel more than 10 movements from 24 weeks).
- Weigh every visit and record, using the same scales.
- Delivery to take place in a consultant unit.
- Plan of care to be documented. Consultant appointments at 16, 28 and 36 weeks.
- Anaesthetic assessment eg sleep apnoea, excessive snoring
- See Physiotherapist if required for example has problems with mobility.
- Serial scans to assess fetal growth (difficult to assess clinically).

Conclusion

It was estimated that at least 360 existing children and 160 live newborn babies lost their mother between 2003-2005 in the last CEMACH study. We know that of these 119 of the women who died were classified as obese (CEMACH 2007a). We also know that approximately 30% of babies who were stillborn or had a neonatal death were born to mothers who had a BMI >30 (CEMACH 2007b) (although caution is urged as there is no national denominator data available).

As midwives we must prepare ourselves for this obesity epidemic and we must be prepared to help women who want to lose weight. Furthermore, we need to dispel the myth that this cannot be achieved safely during in pregnancy. We need to provide practical advice and support to women in a proactive way. This problem will not go away and if we are serious at providing the best care for our women we must start addressing and tackling the problems at the root. This can be achieved by talking to pregnant women about their own weight and the impact that this will have on the future of their children; we generally know obese parents have obese children.

Currently we are using the same BMI for all ethnic groups, this provides a possible explanation why we have increased maternal and perinatal mortality and morbidity in certain ethnic populations. For the future we need to consider the use of culturally adjusted and appropriate BMI as the evidence suggests that the new cut off point for Asians should be a BMI of 25.0.kg/m2 for obesity and 23.0-24.9kg for overweight (Wen et al 2009) as suggested by the WHO criteria.

Most importantly, we need to ensure that the care we give is sensitive and individualised. Safety is vitally important, but key messages and appropriate care will only be accepted by women if they feel empowered and not judged. It is the midwife who is best positioned to offer this safe and comfortable environment.

References

Action on Pre-Eclampsia (www.apec.org.uk) accessed 26.1.10

Barau G, Ribukkard P-Y, Hulsey T.C et al (2006) Linear association beteen maternal pre-pregnancy body mass index and rikd of caesarean secion in term deliveries. *British Journal of Obstetrics and Gynaecology* **113**: 1173–7

Bianco AT, Smilen SW, Davis Y et al (1998) Pregnancy outcome and weight gain recommendations for morbidly obese women. *Obstet Gynecol* **91**: 97–102

Butland B, Jebb S, Kopelman P et al (2007) Foresight Tackling Obesity: Future Choices Project Report http://www.foresight.gov.uk/

Cedergren MI (2004). Maternal morbid obesity and the risk of adverse pregnancy outcome. *Obstetrics & Gynecology* **103**(2): 219–24

Cedergren MI, Kallen BAJ (2003) Maternal obesity and infant heart defects. *Obes Res* **11**: 1065–71

Claesson I, Sydsjo G, Brynhildsen J et al (2007) Weight gain restriction for obese pregnant women: a case-control intervention study DO1: British Journal of Obstetrics and Gynaecology 10.111/j.1471-0528.2007.01531.x

CEMACH (2004) Confidential Enquiry into Maternal and Child Health. Why Mothers Die 2002-2004. The Sixth Report.

CEMACH (2007) Saving Mothers Lives 2003-2005 A report of the UK confidential enquiries into maternal deaths.

CEMACH (2007a) Saving Mothers' Lives Reviewing maternal deaths to make motherhood safer 2003-2005 CEMACH Chiltern Court

CEMACH (2007b) Perinatal mortality 2005 England Wales and Northern Ireland. CEMACH Chiltern Court

Chu SY, Kim SY et al (2007). Maternal obesity and risk of caesarean delivery: a meta-analysis. *Obesity Reviews* **8**(5): 385–94

Department of Health (2005) Delivering Choosing Health Making healthier choices easier. London. http://www.dh.gov.uk/en/Publicationsandstatistics/Publications/PublicationsPolicyAndGuidance/DH_4105355

Department of Health (2007a) Obese Adult Care pathway. http://www.dh.gov.uk/en/Publicationsandstatistics/Publications/PublicationsPolicyAndGuidance

Department of Health (2007b) Raising the issue of weight. http://www.dh.gov.uk/en/Publicationsandstatistics/Publications/PublicationsPolicyAndGuidance/

Despres JP, Lemieux I, Prud'homme D (2001) Treatment of obesity: need to focus on high risk abdominally obese patients. *British Medical Journal* **322:** 716–20

Ehrenberg HM, Mercer BM, Catalano PM (2004) The influence of obesity and diabetes on the prevalence of macrosomia. *American Journal of Obstetrics and Gynecology* **191:** 964–8

Grant I, Fischbacher C, Whyte B (2007) Obesity in Scotland: an epidemiology briefing Scottish Publich Health Observatory. http://www.scotpho.org.uk/home/Publications/scotphoreports/pub_obesityinscotland.asp

Heslehurst N, Ells L, Simpson H et al (2007a) Trends in maternal obesity incidence rates, demographic predictors, and health inequalities in 36 821 women over a 15-year period. *BJOG* **114:** 187–94

Heslehurst N, Lang R, Rankin J, Wilkinson J, Summerbell CD (2007b) Obesity in pregnancy: a study of the impact of maternal obesity on NHS maternity services. *BJOG* **114:** 334–42

Hope J (2007) Obesity is biggest threat to women during pregnancy" *Daily Mail* Accessed Tuesday Dec 4th 2007

Institute of Medicine, editors Rasmussen K.M, YaktineA.L (2009); Committee to Reexamine IOM Pregnancy Weight Guidelines; Institute of Medicine; National Research Council. http://www.nap.edu/catalog/12584.html (assessed October 2009)

Institute of Medicine (1990) Subcommittee on Nutritional Status and Weight Gain During Pregnancy Nutrition during pregnancy Institute of Medicine Washington DC National Academy Press

Jevitt C (2005) Integrating obesity prevention into prenatal care Presentation of finding at the International Conference for Midwifery Brisbane Australia

Jevitt C, Hernadex MS, Groer M (2007) Lactation Complicated by Overweight and Obesity: Supporting the Mother and Newborn. *Journal of Midwifery and Women's*

Health **52**(6): 607–13

Kabiru W, Raynor BD (2004) Obstetric outcomes associated with increase in BMI category during pregnancy. *Am J Obstet Gynecol* **191**(3): 928–32

Kristensen J, Vestergaard M, Wisborg K, Kesmodel U, Secher NJ (2005) Pre-pregnancy weight and the risk of stillbirth and neonatal death. *British Journal of Obstetrics & Gynaecology* **112:** 403–8

National Institute for Health and Clinical Excellence. Antenatal Care: Routine Care for the Healthy Pregnant Woman. London: RCOG, 2008 http://guidance.nice.org.uk/CG62/Guidance/pdf/English (Accessed 26.01.10)

National Audit Office (2001) *Tackling Obesity in England.* The Stationery Office, London

National Health Service Statistics (2006) Statistics on Obesity, Physical Activity and Diet: England, 2006. The Information Centre, Lifestyle Statistics. pregnancy: complications and cost.

National Institute for Health and Clinical Excellence, National Collaborating Centre for Primary Care. Obesity: the Prevention, Identification, Assessment and Management of Overweight and Obesity in Adults and Children. London: NICE; 2006 [www.nice.org.uk/CG043fullguideline]

National Institute for Health and Clinical Excellence, 'Diabetes in pregnancy' Guideline 63 www.nice.org.uk/CG063)

Olafsdottir AS, Skuladottir GV, Thorsdottir I et al (2006) Maternal diet in early and late pregnancy in relation to weight gain. *International Journal of Obesity.* **30**(3): 492–9

O'Toole ML, Sawicki ML, Artal R (2003) Structured diet and physical activity prevent postpartum weight retention. *Journal of womens health* **12:** 991–8

Richens Y (2008) Tackling Maternal Obesity: Suggestions for midwives. *British Journal of Midwifery* **16**(1): 14–9

Royal College of Obstetricans and Gynaecologists (2004) Thromboprophlaxis during pregnancy, labour and after vaginal delivery Green top guideline number 37 [accessed 3-10 2009 http://www.rcog.org.uk/

Royal College of Obstetricans and Gynaecologists Obesity and Reproductive Health - study group statement Consensus views arising from the 53rd Study Group: Obesity and Reproductive Health [accessed 11 December 2007http://www.rcog.org.uk/

Sebire NJ, Jolly M, Harris JP et al (2001) Maternal obesity and pregnancy outcome: a study of 287 213 pregnancies in London. *International Journal of Obesity* **25:** 1175–82

Shaw GM, Todoroff K, Schaffer DM et al (2000) Maternal height and prepregnancy body mass index as risk factors for selected congenital anomalies. *Paediatric and Perinatal Epidemiology* **14**(3): 234–9

Stotland N, Hopkins L Caughey, A (2004) Gestational Weight gain during macrosomia and risk of caesarean birth in nondiabetic nulliparas. *Obtet Gynecol* **104**(4): 1667–77
Stotland NE, Cheng YW, Hopkins LM, Caughey AB (2006) Gestational weight gain

and adverse neonatal outcome among term infants. *Obstetrics and Gynaecology* **108**(3 Pt 1): 635–43

Royal College of Midwives http://www.rcm.org.uk/midwives/news/sharp-rise-in-the-number-of-cases-of-spina-bifida-in-scotland/

Usha Kiran TS, Hemmadi S et al (2005) Outcome of pregnancy in a woman with an increased body mass index. *BJOG* **112**(6): 768–72

Waller DK, Shaw GM, Rasmussen SA et al (2007) Prepregnancy obesity as a risk factor for structural birth defects. *Arch Pediatr Adolesc Med* **161**: 745–50

Watkins M, Ramussen S, Honein M et al (2003) Maternal Obesity and risk for birth defect. *Pediatrics* **111**(5): 1152–8

Weiss JL, Malone FD, Emig D et al (2004) Obesity, obstetric complications and cesarean delivery rate – a population based screening study. *Am J Obstet Gynecol* **190:** 1091–7

Wen CP David Cheng TY, Tsai SP, Chan HT Hsu HL Hsu CC Eriksen MP (2009) Are Asians at greater mortality risks from being overwieght than Caucasians? Redefining obesity for Asains. *Public Health Nurtition* **12**(4) 497-506

Werler MM, Louik C, Shapiro S et al (1996) Prepregnant weight in relation to risk of neural tube defects. *J Am Med Association* **275:** 1089–92

World Health Organisation (1997) Consultation on Obesity Preventing and managing the global epidemic Report on WHO Consultation

WHO expert consultation (2004) Appropriate body-mass index for Asian populations and its implications for policy and intervention strategies. *The Lancet* 157–63

Villamor E, Cnattingius S (2006) Interpregnancy weight change and risk of adverse pregnancy outcomes: a population-based study. *The Lancet* **368:** 1164–70

Zanninoto P, Wardle H, Samakakis E et al (2006) Forecasting obesity to 2010 [accessed December 1st 2007] commissioned by Department of Health. http://www.dh.gov.uk/en/Publicationsandstatistics/Publications/PublicationsStatistics/DH_4138630

Chapter 5

Nutrition in Pregnancy

Carina Venter

Introduction

Dietary intake during pregnancy should provide the required macro and micro nutrients to maintain or improve the health of the pregnant woman and support fetal growth. Pregnancy is a period in the life cycle during which some women may gain unnecessary weight, become overweight, or become obese. Acceptable and recommended weight gain during pregnancy is much debated with no clear guidance in the UK at present. A UK based study indicated that the proportion of obese women at the start of pregnancy has increased from 9.0% to 16.0% over a 15 year period and will be 22% by 2010 if it increases at the current rate (Heslehurst et al 2007a). The author urges in a review of BMI status on obstetric outcomes that national UK guidelines are needed for the management of obese women (Heslehurst et al 2008).

This chapter will discuss nutritional advice during pregnancy to prevent excessive weight gain in all women, with a focus on nutritional advice for women with a raised BMI. Dietary intake during pregnancy not only affects the pregnancy outcome but also has the potential to influence the eating habits and health of the next generation. It is therefore crucial that correct nutritional advice should be given to all pregnant women.

Nutritional assessment

The UK National Institute for Health and Clinical Excellence (NICE) guidelines on Improving the Nutrition of Pregnant and Breastfeeding Mothers and Children in Low-Income Households *(2008)* recommends:
-    *Maternal weight and height should be measured at the booking appointment, and the woman's body mass index should be calculated.*
-    *Repeated weighing during pregnancy should be confined to circumstances in which clinical management is likely to be influenced (see "What is healthy pregnancy weight gain").*

Central to any dietary advice given to pregnant women is the prepregnancy weight, her weight at the initial appointment, and her body mass index (BMI). This will determine how much weight should be gained during pregnancy and the amount of energy required from the pregnancy diet.

Determining BMI

The BMI (Thomas and Bishop 2007) score is the standard marker for describing obesity in populations. Body Mass Index uses a mathematical formula that takes into account both a person's height and weight. Body Mass Index equals a person's weight (in kilograms) divided by height (in meters) squared:

$$\text{weight [kg] / height [m]}^2.$$

Adults

The BMI value for adults should be interpreted using the prepregnancy weight or weight at the initial assessment. This is classified as:

- <16 Severely underweight
- 16 – 19 Underweight
- 20 – 25 Normal range
- 26 – 30 Overweight
- 31 – 40 Obese
- >40 Morbidly obese.

See *Table 5.1* for the World Health Organisation (WHO) classification of the BMI.

Teenagers

For children and young people (those aged <18 years), BMI is not a static measurement. It varies from birth to adulthood and is different between boys and girls. Interpretation of BMI values in children and young people therefore depends on using BMI percentiles (Thomas and Bishop 2007a). For clinical use, obese children are those with a BMI ≥98th centile of the UK 1990 reference chart for age and sex.

Table 5.1: BMI classification according to the WHO (DH 2007)	
Classification	**BMI(kg/m2) Principal cut-off points**
Underweight	less than 18.50
Severe thinness	less than 16.00
Moderate thinness	16.00 - 16.99
Mild thinness	17.00 - 18.49
Normal Range	18.50 - 24.99
Overweight	greater than or equal to 25.00
Pre-obese	25.00 - 29.99
Obese	greater than or equal to 30.00
Obese class I	30.00 - 34.99
Obese class II	35.00 - 39.99
Obese class III	greater than or equal to 40.00

What is healthy pregnancy weight gain?

Olson (2008) suggests that to some extent, weight gain during pregnancy will affect:

- infant size at birth
- pregnancy, labour, and delivery complications
- neonatal, infant, and child outcomes
- maternal weight and health outcomes.

Weight gain during pregnancy accounts for increased blood volume, maternal tissue (womb, placenta, breasts), amniotic fluid, fluid retention, maternal fat and nutrient stores and the weight of the baby.

There are no official recommendations in the UK for weight gain during pregnancy. Maternal dietary intake should be sufficient to sustain a healthy pregnancy. However, excess weight gain during pregnancy has health implications for both the mother and baby and may result in retention of weight gain after the baby is born, particularly with early cessation of breastfeeding (Williamson et al 1994).

In the early 1900s, most medical authorities recommended a weight gain of less than 9.1 kg (Feig and Naylor 1998). This was mainly due to the adverse affects seen of higher weight gain on maternal weight gain, fetal macrosomia and problems during delivery (Thorsdottir et al 2002). However by the 1970s, women were being encouraged to gain at least 11.4 kg (Feig and Naylor 1998) as insufficient weight gain could contribute to premature births and to low birth weight term infants.

In 1990, the Institute of Medicine USA (IOM) made recommendations regarding pregnancy weight gain (*Table 5.2*) that was associated with better pregnancy outcomes.

These guidelines aim to achieve an optimal infant birth weight of between 3000 and 4000 grams (g), the birth weights in the United States associated with the lowest risk of mortality (Olson 2008). Although these guidelines were questioned by Feig and Naylor (1998), it has been accepted by the American Dietetic Association (ADA) (2008) and supported by a landmark systematic review in 2000 (Abrams et al 2000). In addition, Olson et al (2008) conclude in a recent review that the IOM recommendations lead to better pregnancy outcome with the possible exception of very obese women, who may benefit from weight gains less than the 7 kg recommended.

Table 5.2 IOM 1990 and ADA recommendations for weight gain during pregnancy (American Dietetic Association 2008)

Body Mass Index	Recommended Weight Gain	Weight Gain/Week After 12 Weeks
<19.8	12.5 to 18 kg (28-40 lb)	0.5 kg (1 lb)
19.6-26.0	11.5 to 16 kg (25-35 lb)	0.4 kg (0.88 lb)
26.0 to 29.0	7 to 11.5 kg (15-25 lb)	0.3 kg (0.66 lb)
>29.0	At least 7.0 kg (15 lb)	
Twin pregnancy	15.9 – 20.4 kg (34 – 45 lb)	0.7 kg
Triplet pregnancy	Overall gain of 22.7 kg (50 lb)	

Young adolescents (<2 years after menarche) and African American women should strive for gains at the upper end of the range. Short women (<62 inches or <157 centimetres) should strive for gains at the lower end of the range.

Weight gain for all women

Frederick et al (2008) found a 76% increased risk of delivering a macrosomic infant (≥4000 g) among women who gained more weight in pregnancy than the IOM recommends, adjusting for prepregnancy BMI. This indicates that in all BMI groups, it is paramount not to gain more weight than the top range indicates. A large Swedish study (Cedergren 2006) also indicated that gaining more than 16 kg (35.2 pounds) increased the risk of pre-eclampsia and caesarean delivery in women of all weight ranges. However, gaining less than 8 kg (17.6 pounds) decreased the risk of pre eclampsia in all but the underweight women. A decreased risk of caesarean delivery was also seen in women with a BMI ≥25 (overweight and obese) who gained less than 8 kg.

Looking at infant outcomes vs. maternal weight gain, Frederick et al (2008) found a 76% increased risk of delivering a macrosomic infant (≥4000 g) among women who gained more weight in pregnancy than the IOM recommends made in 1990, adjusting for pre-pregnancy BMI.This data indicates that in all BMI groups, it is paramount not to gain more weight than the top range indicated by the IOM. In addition, Stotland et al (2006) found that gestational weight gain above the IOM 1990 guidelines was associated with a low 5-minute Apgar score, assisted ventilation, seizure, hypoglycaemia, polycythemia, meconium aspiration syndrome, and large for gestational age (LGA) infants compared with women within weight gain guidelines. Gestational weight gain below the IOM 1990 guidelines was associated with decreased odds of neonatal intensive care unit admission, increased risk of seizure, general hospital stay of more than 5 days and increased odds of small for date (SFD) deliveries.

In summary, gaining more weight than indicated by the IOM in 1990 (more than the top range for each BMI category or >16-18 kg) is associated with unwanted pregnancy outcomes for both the mother and infant. Gaining less than 7-8 kg of weight may decrease the risk of PE and the need for a caesarean section but could be outweighed by longer hospital stay, infant seizures and SFD babies.

Weight gain in underweight and normal weight women

Low weight gain in underweight and normal weight women can lead to low birth weight (LBW) infants (Goldberg 2003). In a population based cohort study of normal weight women between the ages of 18 and 35 years, DeVader et al (2007) showed that gaining within the IOM recommendations (11.5-16 kg) is associated with the lowest risk of bearing a SFD or LGA infant. In support of this, Rode et al (2007) showed in normal BMI women that a weight gain less than the IOM 1990 recommendations increased the risk for a baby weighing less than 3 kg, and weight gain more than the IOM recommendations increased the risk for a baby weighing more than 4 kg.

Beyond the effect on birth weight, two studies (DeVader et al 2007; Thorsdottir et al 2002) found that among normal BMI pregnant women, gaining less weight than the IOM 1990 recommendations was associated with decreased prevalence of PE, cephalopelvic disproportion, failed induction, and caesarean delivery compared with gaining within the recommended range. Among women who gained more than the IOM 1990 recommends there was increased prevalence of PE, cephalopelvic disproportion, failed induction, and caesarean delivery compared to the reference group.

Weight gain in overweight or obese women

Despite the ADA and IOM 1990 recommendations, which some have been questioned to be too liberal, many women still exceed them. Women who are overweight before pregnancy are most vulnerable to excessive gestational weight gain. During the postpartum period, 14% to 20% of women may retain weight from pregnancy, which elevates risk of later health problems for both the mother and infant (Walker 2007). In particular, excess weight gain during pregnancy is associated with the child being overweight at 3 years, and this effect is greater in mothers with increased BMI (Olson et al 2008). Maternal weight gain during pregnancy could therefore play an important role in the rise seen in childhood obesity in the UK. Almost a fifth of 2 to 5 year olds are now obese, while a further 14% are overweight (Cross Government Obesity Unit, Department of Health [DH] and Department for Children 2008).

Two studies (Rode et al 2007; Schieve et al 1998) found that the relationships between gestational weight gain and birth weight was less apparent in overweight and obese women. Olson (2008) concludes that very obese women may benefit from weight gains less than the 7 kg recommended. Kiel et al (2007) provided the answer regarding ideal weight gain in overweight/obese women in a study of 120 251 women in the USA who gave birth to term singletons between 1990-2001. The study demonstrated that gestational weight gain for overweight or obese pregnant women of less than the currently recommended 7 kg was associated with a significantly lower risk of PE, caesarean delivery, and LGA birth. On the other hand, gaining less than the recommended weight also increased the risk of SFD births. Kiel et al. showed that the following pattern of weight gain lead to improved infant outcomes:

Table 5.3: New IOM recommendations for total and rate of weight gain during pregnancy (Institute of Medicine 2009)

Prepregnancy BMI	BMI+ (kg/m2) (WHO)	Total Weight Gain Range (lbs)	Rates of Weight Gain* 2nd and 3rd Trimester (Mean Range in kg/wk)	Rates of WeightGain* 2nd and 3rd Trimester (Mean Range in lbs/wk)
Underweight	<18.5	12.7 to 18.2 kg (28–40 lbs)	450 g (450-590 g)	1(1–1.3)
Normal weight	18.5-24.9	11.4 to 15.9 kg (25-35lbs)	450 g (360-450 g)	1(0.8–1)
Overweight	25.0-29.9	6.8 to 11.4 kg (15–25 lbs)	270 g (230–320 g)	0.6(0.5–0.7)
Obese (includes all classes)	≥30.0	5 – 9 kg (11–20 lbs)	230 g (180– 270 g)	0.5(0.4– 0.6)

* Calculations assume a 0.5–2 kg (1.1–4.4 lbs) weight gain in the first trimester

- weight gain of 4.55–11.36 kg for women with a BMI of 30.0–34.9
- weight gain of 0–4.09 kg for women with a BMI of 35.0–39.9
- weight loss of 0–4.09 kg for women with a BMI ≥40

Similarly, Cedergren et al (2006) reflected these finding, reporting that a low pregnancy weight gain (<8 kg) was associated with decreased risk of caesarean delivery in women with a BMI ≥25 (overweight and obese).

Based on all these studies, the IOM guidelines have been updated very recently(Institute of Medicine 2009) (*Table 5.3*). In these latest guidelines, they have adjusted the BMI ranges and the recommended weight gain in obese women.

Weight gain in teenagers

The optimal weight gain for pregnant teenagers is uncertain. Rees et al (1992) indicated that a weight gain of 0.6 kg/week increases the likelihood of having a baby with a normal weight of between 3-4 kg. Heari et al (2009) showed that obese teens were at higher risk of caesarean delivery and gestational diabetes than normal weight teens and concluded that both overweight and obese teens were at higher risk of adverse pregnancy outcomes.

Nutrition advice during pregnancy

As discussed, nutrition advice during pregnancy used to focus on sufficient weight gain to prevent under nutrition and LBW babies (Bruce and Tchabo 1989; Orstead et al 1985). Nowadays however, attention is focused on reducing overconsumption/overweight and health risks to the infant and mother. Moreover, overconsumption/overweight during pregnancy does not guarantee adequacy of critical nutrients (i.e. against birth defects or for brain development).

The role of the health care professional (HCP) in conveying dietary advice during pregnancy is very important. It is known that women's gestational weight gains tend to follow the recommendations of HCPs (Olson 2008). Stotland et al (2006) indicated in a USA study that only a third of pregnant women were given nutrition advice and that 50% were given the wrong advice regarding weight gain. Heslehurst et al (2007b) performed a qualitative study on maternity services in the North East of England showing that dietary information to patients was an issue, with the NHS patient information booklet the only form of dietary patient information in the majority of maternity units. This booklet generally addresses healthy and safe eating rather than weight gain or specific dietary requirements related to BMI. Midwives stated that dietary information given to pregnant women was inconsistent and on an *ad hoc* basis and none of the midwifery units had a policy or guideline on recommended weight gain during pregnancy. Some units recommended weight stability rather than weight gain in obese women. A few maternity units mentioned that a new policy for maternal obesity/nutrition was under development. Most maternity units felt that they needed better links with dietitians, more information to give detailed dietary advice, time to explain the risks of being obese or gaining too much weight, or community interventions prior to becoming pregnant, but realised the problems regarding limited resources. In addition, midwives also felt it was difficult to address the issue of obesity with pregnant women as "women do not like to be told they are overweight".

Six studies (Absee et al 2009, Claesson et al 2008; Kinnunen et al 2007; Olson et al 2004; Polley et al 2002; Wolff et al 2008) are cited in the literature and address the issue of excessive maternal weight gain during pregnancy (*Table 5.4*).

Table 5.4 Clinical intervention studies on promoting healthy pregnancy weight gains – adapted from (Olson 2008)

Author (Reference)	Design	Population and sample	Intervention	Details of dietary intervention	Weight outcome
Polley et al. (2002)	Randomized controlled trial	Low-income women receiving prenatal care at a hospital-based clinic in a large U.S. city 61 normal BMI (30 l) 49 overweight BMI (27 l); black and white women	Stepped-care behavioural intervention; education about weight gain, healthy eating and exercise; individual graphs for weight gain	HCP involved: master's and doctoral level staff with training in nutrition or clinical psychology. The primary focus: decreasing high-fat foods and substituting healthier alternatives If these approaches did not help then a more structured meal plan and individualized calorie goals were added. Support provided between visits. Exercise intervention: walking and developing a more active lifestyle.	Normal BMI women: % with excessive gain reduced from 58% to 33% (p<0.05) Overweight BMI: % with excessive gain increased from 32% to 59% (p = 0.09)
Olson et al. (2004)	Prospective cohort with historical control group	Rural primarily white U.S. women 421 normal BMI (131 l) 139 overweight BMI	Health care provider monitoring of weight gain	"Health Checkbook" with information on weight gain and diet-self monitoring tools.	Significant effect in low-income women only (p<0.05) (see below)

Table 5.4 Clinical intervention studies on promoting healthy pregnancy weight gains – adapted from (Olson 2008)

(48 1)				Ongoing support provided with newsletters by mail with return postcards for goal setting.	Normal BMI women:% with excessive gain reduced from 45% to 29% (p<0.05) Overweight BMI:% with excessive gain reduced from 72% to 44% (p<0.05)
Kinnunen et al. (2007),	Selected intervention (N = 3) and control maternity clinics (N = 3)	Finnish women, primaparous 49 intervention 56 control 75% and 79% normal BMI (respectively)	Individual counselling on: Weight gain Physical activity–one primary and four boosters Diet–one primary and three boosters	Health care professional involved: Public health nurses. Following provided: - Regular meal pattern, - Five portions of fruit and vegetables - High fibre bread - Restrict the intake of high-sugar snacks to 1 portion per day Dietary counselling: one primary counselling session at 16–18 weeks' gestation visit and three booster sessions until the 37th gestation week. A food frequency	No significant effect on% exceeding IOM 46% in intervention and 30% in control Significant differences in diet

Table 5.4 Clinical intervention studies on promoting healthy pregnancy weight gains – adapted from (Olson 2008)

Claesson et al. (2008)	Prospective case control (intervention and comparison cities)	Obese (BMI ≥30) healthy Swedish women 155 intervention 193 control	Patient education Women offered individual, weekly 30-minute motivational interviews	HCP involved: a specially trained midwife. Motivational interview/ talk in early pregnancy regarding change of behaviour. • Assessment of the pregnant woman's knowledge of risk obesity during pregnancy and questionnaire was used to assess food intake. Need for change discussed and healthy diet leaflets provided. Food diaries kept and discussed. Exercise intervention: a minimum of 30 min of moderate-intensity physical activity on 5 weekdays for health and a minimum of 40 min of high-intensity physical activity three times per week for fitness.	Significant effect on weight gain <7 kg (p = 0.003) 35.7% in intervention and 20.5% in control gained <7 kg

Table 5.4 Clinical intervention studies on promoting healthy pregnancy weight gains – adapted from (Olson 2008)

			provision of information. • Food and eating behaviour was assessed and written information provided. • Weekly follow-up Exercise intervention: Aqua aerobics once or twice per week	
Wolff et al. (2008)	Randomized controlled trial	Obese (BMI ≥30) non-diabetic, non-smoking Danish women 23 intervention 27 control	10 one-hour consultations with dietitian to achieve energy restriction per Danish macronutrient guidelines	HCP involved: Trained dietitian 10 consultations of 1 h each with a trained dietitian during the pregnancy. Healthy diet according to the official Danish dietary recommendations (fat intake 30%, protein intake: 15–20%, carbohydrate intake: 50–55%). The energy intake was individually estimated energy requirements and estimated energetic cost of fetal growth Food diaries kept, analysed and	Significant difference in energy intake in expected direction (p = 0.001) Significant effect on weight gain (6.6 kg in intervention versus 13.3 kg in control; p = 0.002)

Table 5.4 Clinical intervention studies on promoting healthy pregnancy weight gains – adapted from (Olson 2008)

Asbee et al. (2009)	Randomized controlled trial	USA women who presented age 18–49 years, English-speaking, Spanish-speaking, or both, and singleton pregnancy. A total of 100 women were randomized to the study (lifestyle counseling 57, routine prenatal care 43).	Group 1: underweight and normal-weight (BMI less than 26). Group 2: overweight (BMI between 26 and 30). Group 3: obese (BMI higher than 30). Patients were assigned randomly to either the control group (pregnancy booklet), who received routine prenatal care for the remainder of the pregnancy, or to the intervention group, who received the standardized protocol of dietary and lifestyle counselling.	discussed. Exercise intervention: None. HCP involved: registered dietitian. Information on Pregnancy-specific dietary and lifestyle choices. Patient-focused caloric value divided in a 40% carbohydrate, 30% protein, and 30% fat fashion. Exercise intervention: moderate-intensity exercise at least three times per week and preferably five times per week.	Significant effect on weight gain (28.7_12.5 lb in active compared with 35.6_15.5 lb in control, P_.01). More caesarean deliveries due to "failure to progress" (routine prenatal care 58.3% compared with lifestyle counselling 25.0%, P_.02). Patients who did not adhere to the IOM guidelines had significantly heavier neonates (adherent 3,203.2_427.2 g compared with not adherent 3,517.4_572.4 g, $P<.01$).

HCP, Health Care Professional; BMI, body mass index; I, intervention; IOM, Institute of Medicine.

These studies show the importance of detailed dietary advice and need for continuous support to be given to pregnant women, as well as the important role of HCPs such as a dietitian and midwife. Nutrition advice should also address psychological factors and access to healthy food as it is known that women from disadvantaged groups have a poorer diet and are more likely to be obese or to show low weight gain during pregnancy (Gibson 2006; NICE 2008). A thorough assessment and discussion of BMI and the consequences of being overweight or obese is also important as women often underestimate their true weight status and this increases their likelihood of unnecessary weight gain during pregnancy. They are often not informed of the risks (Herring et al 2008; Strychar et al 2000).

The NICE (2008) guidelines recommend that the following nutrition information should be given to pregnant women:

1) At the first contact with a healthcare professional:

● Folic acid supplementation recommendations should be provided. Women should be advised to take 400 micrograms (µg) folic acid daily before pregnancy and throughout the first 12 weeks of pregnancy, even if they are already eating foods fortified with folic acid or rich in folate.

● Food hygiene information, including how to reduce the risk of a food acquired infection

2) At booking (ideally by 10 weeks):

● Nutrition and diet advice; eating adequate amounts of fruit, vegetables and oily fish, and taking the appropriate supplement including folic acid and vitamin D

● Exercise advice; women should be encouraged to do a brisk walk or other moderate exercise for at least 30 minutes on at least 5 days of the week) and to do their pelvic floor exercises.

The guidelines also recommends to obstetricians, gynaecologists, GPs, midwives, health visitors, nurses, dietitians, those working in contraceptive services or on weight management programmes (commercial or voluntary) who identify pregnant women who have a prepregnancy BMI>30, and those with a BMI>30 who have a baby or who may become pregnant, that:

1) They inform their patients that increased weight poses risks to themselves and their babies.
2) They should encourage them to lose weight before becoming pregnant or after pregnancy.

They should also:

● Provide a structured programme addressing why women find it difficult to lose weight and is tailored to the needs of the individual or group.
● Provide healthy eating advice.

- Recommend 30 min of exercise (brisk walk) 5 times per week.
- Identify barriers to change and provide ongoing support.
- Refer these women to a dietitian for assessment and advice.
- Advise that weight loss is not recommended.

Energy intake

The nutritional requirements of pregnancy must be met by dietary intake and maternal body stores. It is well known that fetal growth depends on the nutritional status and intake of the mother before and during pregnancy. The nutrient supply to the fetus is regulated by:
- Changes in maternal food choice and dietary intake
- Maternal metabolic adaptation
- Altered maternal absorption
- Fetal uptake
- Varying maternal uptake. (Thomas and Bishop 2007b)

Recommended intake

The actual amount of energy needed will vary from person to person and depends on their basal metabolic rate and their level of activity. Although it is not expected of midwives to calculate energy requirements and give detailed dietary advice, the next section aims to give the midwife a better understanding of assessing nutritional intake.

Calculation energy requirements for females in the UK

In order to calculate energy requirements according to the DH (1991), the woman's height, ideal body weight and age should be known. This information can ve provided by a qualified dietician. Firstly, the basal metabolic rate (BMR) is calculated. This is then adjusted for activity level in order to calculate the estimated energy requirements.

1) BMR is calculated using the following equation:

BMR for females 10-17 years = 13.4 x weight (kg) + 692
BMR for females 18-29 years = 14.8 x weight (kg) + 487
BMR for females 30-59 years = 8.3 x weight (kg) + 846

2) Estimated energy requirements = BMR x activity factor

For example:
Female 25 years old, recommended weight range (50–62 kg: average 56 kg) and she is inactive:

Estimated energy requirements:
14.8 x 56 kg + 487 x 1.4 = 1842 kcal

Energy requirements during pregnancy:

The total energy cost of pregnancy has been estimated between 70000 and 76000 kcal (DH 1991). This additional energy need is estimated to be:
- 20 kcal/day in the first trimester
- 85 kcal/day in the second trimester
- 310 kcal/day in the third trimester. (Thomas and Bishop 2007b)

However, the DH (1991) recommends that during the first two trimesters of pregnancy, there is no need for additional energy; only an additional 200 kcal per day (*Table 5.5 and Table 5.6*) is needed in the third trimester. Their recommendations are based on the fact that possible hormonal adaptations and reduced activity during pregnancy may not necessitate the need for any additional energy. This is lower than the recommendation by the ADA (2008) which advises an increase of 300 kcal per day in the second trimester and 300 kcal to 500 kcal per day in the third trimester. This additional energy intake during pregnancy is needed for the following:

Table 5.5 Activity level		
Inactive	Assume sitting most of the day with less than 2 hours on their feet.	1.4
Light	Assume some daily exercise – at work or tasks about the house or garden – with at least 2 hours on their feet.	1.5
Moderate	Assume 6 hours on their feet or regular strenuous exercise	1.64
Heavy	Those in heavy labouring jobs	1.82

- Growth of the fetus
- Breast tissue development
- Maternal stores of 2-2.4 kg
- Increased blood flow.

In order to allow for the pregnancy needs in the last trimester, 200 kcal should be added.

Looking back at the previously used example, energy needs during the last trimester of pregnancy for this individual will be:
1842 + 200 kcal = 2042 kcal

In clinical dietetic practice, the calculated energy requirements will be divided into the five foods groups which are:

Table 5.6 What does 200 kcal look like?

500 ml Coca Cola	I small sweet muffin
6-7 Baby Carrots	½ bagel (70 g)
3 large slices Honeydew Melon	2 small wheat dinner rolls (66 g)
2 Apples	2 ½ slices bread
I bunch (290 g) Grapes	145 g Cooked Pasta
12 dried apricots	60 ml cream liqueur
I medium avocado	41 g Snickers Chocolate Bar
I large glass Whole Milk	57 g "Smarties" type confectionery
200 g Low fat Strawberry Yogurt	54 g jelly bean type confectionery
100 g All Bran	56 g fruit pie
55 g crunchy type cereal	53 g Brown Sugar
54 g Puffed Rice Cereal	¾ doughnut (52 g)
½ beef burger (75 g)	50 g salted crackers
75 g French fries	52 g Salted Pretzels
35 g Almonds/mixed nuts	41 g Doritos
51 g Medium Cheddar Cheese	37 g crisps
I large hot dog (wiener)	28 g butter
200 g Sliced Smoked Turkey/ham	23 g oil
3 eggs	
½ can Tuna Packed in Oil	

- Bread, cereal and potatoes
- Fruit and vegetables
- Milk, cheese and yoghurt
- Meat, fish and vegetarian alternatives
- Fats and sugars.

Finally, the portion sizes are quantified into portions of food.

For example: A woman with a height of 1.65 m has a recommended/ideal weight range of 50.4-68 kg (average 59 kg) and will require a kcal intake of 2000 in the first two trimesters and 2200 kcal in the third trimester *(Table 5.7)*. When dealing with obese pregnant teenagers, it is suggested that the help and support of a dietitian is requested due to the complexity of supporting growth of both the mother and fetus, while preventing further excessive weight gain.

Protein

The optimal amount of protein required during pregnancy is not known. It is suggested that both adult and teenage females should consume an additional 6g of protein during pregnancy to allow for the growth of the fetus and growth/maintenance of maternal tissue (DH 1991).

Recommendations

The recommended nutrient intake (RNI) for protein during pregnancy for both adult and teenage females are 45g + 6g = 51g protein per day (Department of Health (DH) 1991).
Adults and teenage females should therefore aim to consume at least 45g + 6g = 51g protein per day (DH 1991).

Fat

There are no official recommendations regarding the intake of fat during pregnancy. However, the importance of omega-3 fatty acids in neural and cognitive development (Cetin and Koletzko 2008) and allergy prevention (Dunstan et al 2003) has been highlighted. Omega-3 fatty acids belong to the group of poly unsaturated fatty acids.

Table 5.7 Sample menu based on a 2000 kcal diet

	Portions	
Breakfast	2 Bread, cereal, potato, pasta	6 tablespoons cereal fortified with iron and folic acid
	1 Milk and dairy	200 ml semi-skimmed milk
	1 Fruit and vegetable	150 ml orange juice
		Hot beverage
Snack	1 Bread, cereal, potato	½ large bagel
	1 fat and sugar/extras	1 tsp butter/spread
	1 milk and dairy	1-2 oz hard cheese
	1 Fruit and vegetable	1 heaped tablespoon of raisins
Noon Meal	2 Bread, cereal, potato, pasta	Sandwich with 2 slices bread, 2 oz lunch meat, lettuce, tomato,
	Meat, fish and alternatives	mustard, mayonnaise (1 tsp)
	1 Fruit and vegetable	and spread (2tsp)
	3 fats and sugar/extras	
	1 Fruit and vegetable	Fresh apple
	1 milk and dairy	200 ml semi-skimmed milk
Snack	1 Fruit and vegetable	150 ml cup tomato or vegetable juice
Evening Meal	Meat, fish and alternatives	2 oz roast beef or salmon
	2 Bread, cereal, potato, pasta	4 tablespoons mashed potato or brown rice
	1 Fruit and vegetable	3 heaped tablespoons of broccoli or Brussels sprouts
	1 Fruit and vegetable	1 side salad with salad dressing
	1 fat and sugar/extra	(1 tsp)
	1 Fruit and vegetable	1 Sliced peach with whipped
	1 fat and sugar/extras	topping (2tsp)
Snack	1 Bread, cereal, potato	2-3 crackers or wholemeal crispbread
	2 fats and sugar/extras	1 tsp butter/spread and 1 tsp jam

Note: Additional water should be consumed throughout the day.

Recommendations

The dietary reference values (DRV) for these fats are 6% of the total fat intake per day and should not exceed 10%. No specific recommendations for omega-3 fatty acids exist either. However, The Associate Parliamentary Food and Health Forum (2007) published the Links Between Diet and Behaviour report that recommended that pregnant and lactating women should aim to achieve an average daily intake of at least 1000 mg of omega-3 fatty acids of which 200mg/day should be docosahexanoic acid, the fatty acid important for cognitive development. No recommendations regarding eicospentanoic acid intake (which plays an important role in allergy prevention) exist. Omega-3 fatty acids are naturally found in salmon, sardines, pilchards, mackerel, kipper, huss/dogfish and crab; as well as linseed or flax seed.

Due to the mercury content of oily fish, the Food Standards Agency (2009a) recommends the following regarding fish intake during pregnancy:

> *Avoid eating shark, swordfish and marlin. And limit the amount of tuna you eat to no more than two steaks a week (weighing about 140g cooked or 170g raw) or four medium size cans a week (about 140g drained weight per can). This is because of the levels of mercury in these fish. At high levels, mercury can harm a baby's developing nervous system.*
> *Have no more than two portions of oily fish a week. Oily fish includes fresh tuna (not canned tuna), mackerel, sardines and trout.*

If pregnant women choose to take an omega-3 supplement during pregnancy, it is important to choose fish oil, rather than cod liver oil supplements. This is due to the high vitamin A content of fish liver oils (Thomas and Bishop 2007b).

A number of vitamins and minerals are of particular importance during pregnancy and are discussed below. Special care should be taken to ensure sufficient intake of these nutrients in teenage girls.

Folate

Folic acid supplementation when women are planning for a pregnancy and during the first 12 weeks of pregnancy is recommended for the prevention of neural tube defects and megaloblastic anaemia (DH 1991, Thomas and Bishop 2007b). Women's diets typically provide about 250ug folate/day (Henderson et al 2003)

Recommendations

A daily supplement of 400ug folic acid should be taken. A bigger dose of folic acid will be needed for women who:
- have had an infant with spina bifida
- are taking medication for epilepsy
- are diabetic
- have coeliac disease.

Good sources include broccoli, Brussels sprouts, asparagus, peas, chickpeas and brown rice. Other useful sources include fortified breakfast cereals, some bread and fruit, such as oranges and bananas (Food Standards Agency 2009b).

Vitamin A

During pregnancy, vitamin A is needed for growth of the fetus and maternal tissue. However, an intake above 3300 ug/day could be teratogenic and pregnant women or women who plan to get pregnant are therefore recommended not to eat liver or take supplements containing vitamin A (DH 1991).

Recommendations

The RNI of 600 ug vitamin A per day increases for women of all ages (11-50+ years) by 100 ug leading to a RNI of 700 ug vitamin A per day. Dietary sources of vitamin A include leafy dark green vegetables, orange vegetables and fruits, and tomatoes and tomato products. Beta-carotene is the precursor of vitamin A and non-toxic/non-teratogenic (DH 1991).

Iron and Vitamin C

The fetus accumulates most of its iron from the mother's reserves during the last trimester. The iron requirements needed to support a full term pregnancy is 680 mg. Most women of childbearing age should have sufficient iron stores to provide iron to the fetus. This process is assisted by cessation of menstruation, mobilisation of maternal stores and increased intestinal absorption. There are however some concerns such as:
- Women who usually experience high menstrual losses may need more

iron than the recommended DRV and may therefore need supplementation (DH 1991).

- Data from the National Diet and Nutrition Survey in 2003 indicated that more than 40% of 19-64 year old women in the UK consume less than the lower recommended intake (Henderson et al 2003).

Recommendations

The RNI for iron for females 11-64 years is 14.8 mg per day with no recommended increase during pregnancy (DH 1991). Iron is found in animal (meat, poultry and fish) and plant sources (green vegetables). Iron from animal sources (haem iron) is better absorbed than iron from plant sources (non-haem iron). Phytate (in cereals and pulses), fibre, tannins (in tea) and calcium reduces the absorption of iron.

The RNI of vitamin C is increased by 10 mg in the last trimester of

Table 5.8 Non-dairy sources of calcium (Wright and Meyer 2009)	
100g sardines (tinned - where bones eaten)	500mg
40g dry instant porridge (before milk added)	480mg
50g tofu (soya bean curd)	255mg
1 glass/200mls calcium enriched soya milk	250mg
1 glass/200mls calcium fortified orange juice	245mg
1 glass/200mls calcium enriched oat milk	240mg
1 glass/200mls calcium enriched soya fruit drink	240mg
100g muesli = 1 large bowl	200mg
3 dried figs	170mg
100g spinach	160mg
125g soya yogurt	125mg
2 heaped tablespoon red kidney beans	100mg
100g = 3 slices white bread	100mg
30g breakfast cereals	100mg

Most importantly: "Eating for two" does not mean eating for two. Portion control may be needed for some women to prevent unnecessary weight gain.

pregnancy for all women to 50 mg per day (DH 1991). Vitamin C (peppers, strawberries, oranges, tomatoes, broccoli and Brussels sprouts) assists with the absorption non-haem iron when eaten at the same time. The same applies to meat, fish and poultry. Fortified breakfast cereal and bread also act as valuable sources of iron. Particular attention should be paid to ensure adequate intake of vitamin C by female smokers (Haste et al 1990). In some cases iron supplementation will be prescribed following guidelines and the clinicians' discretion.

Calcium and Vitamin D

The increased requirements for calcium are mostly met by the increased absorption seen during pregnancy due to hormonal changes. There are however some women who may be at risk of consuming insufficient amounts of calcium such as those with allergies/intolerances to dairy, women who do not like the taste of dairy foods, teenage mothers or those consuming a high fibre diet, and especially Asian women who may also have a low vitamin D status (NICE 2008).

Recommendations

The RNI's for calcium for females aged 15-18 years (800 mg) and females aged 19-50 years (700mg) also apply to pregnant women in those age groups (DH 1991). The report also recommends all pregnant women should receive supplementary vitamin D to achieve an intake of 10 ug/day.

The best dietary sources of calcium are milk and milk products and recommended portions per day are suggested in *Table 5.7*. For non-dairy sources of calcium see *Table 5.8*.

Vitamin D is usually obtained during exposure to sunlight, but not when sunscreens with a very high factor are used (Peacey et al 2006). Dietary sources include vitamin D enriched spreads, cheese, fatty/oily fish and eggs (Thomas and Bishop 2007b).

Zinc

Extra zinc is required during pregnancy, especially during the last trimester However the DH (1991) recommends that no extra zinc is required during pregnancy. This is due to metabolic adaptations ensuring sufficient transfer of zinc to the fetus when adhering to the RNI.

Recommendation

The RNI for zinc is 7 mg/day (females 15 to 50+ years) and also applies to pregnant women. Foods high in zinc include seafood, milk, liver, oatmeal, whole corn, wheat germ, yeast, meat, fish, eggs and green leafy vegetables.

Alcohol intake during pregnancy

Pregnant women and women planning a pregnancy should be advised to avoid drinking alcohol in the first 3 months of pregnancy if possible because it may be associated with an increased risk of miscarriage. If women choose to drink alcohol during pregnancy they should be advised to drink no more than 1 to 2 units once or twice a week. In the UK, 1 unit equals half a pint of ordinary strength lager or beer, or 1 shot [25 ml] of spirits. For wine drinkers, 1 small glass [125 ml] is equal to 1.5 UK units (NICE 2008).

Although there is uncertainty regarding a safe level of alcohol consumption in pregnancy, at this low level there is no evidence of harm to the unborn baby. Women should be informed that getting drunk or binge drinking during pregnancy (defined as more than 5 standard drinks or 7.5 UK units on a single occasion) may be harmful to the unborn baby.

Nutritional recommendations for multiple pregnancies

The ADA recommends that women carrying more than one baby have increased needs for energy, folate, omega-3 fatty acids, iron, calcium and vitamin D. However, the DH does not give additional recommendations for any nutrients in multiple pregnancies.

Healthy eating during pregnancy

Healthy eating during pregnancy can be summarised in *Table 5.9*

Previously, the UK Government advised that where anyone in a child's immediate family had a known allergy, mothers may wish to avoid eating peanuts during pregnancy, whilst breastfeeding, and to delay introducing peanut into the diet of these children until three years of age. This was precautionary advice that was issued in 1998 based on a concern related to the evidence base available at that time, that consumption of peanut by the mother could, in theory, transfer through to the developing infant and affect whether or not they develop peanut allergy.

Table 5.9 Summary of healthy eating during pregnancy

Do eat: A healthy balanced diet from all five food groups
Regular meals and snacks.

Do drink: Sufficient amounts of fluids, preferably water and other non-caffienated drinks.

Do take: A folic acid supplement for the first 12 weeks and continue with intake of folate rich foods.

Do follow: Strict food safety and hygiene guidelines (*Table 5.10*)

Be careful: Follow guidelines regarding intake of :
- Fatty fish/oily fish
- Alcohol
- Caffeine (less than 300 mg per day) (*Table 5.11*)

Avoid: Liver and liver products as well as vitamin A supplementation
All other foods implicated in food safety.

This advice has now been withdrawn and the current advice from the Food Standards Agency and the Committee on Toxicity of Chemicals in Food states that if mothers would like to eat peanuts or foods containing peanuts during pregnancy or breastfeeding, then they can choose to do so as part of a healthy balanced diet, irrespective of whether their child has a family history of allergies (Committee on Toxicity of Chemicals in Food 2009).

Table 5.10 Food safety and hygiene (Thomas & Bishop 2007b)

To avoid toxoplasma infection which can cause foetal abnormalities such as mental retardation and blindness:

- Cook all meat and poultry thoroughly.
- Wash fruit, vegetables and salads to remove all traces of soil.

To avoid salmonella infection which can trigger premature labour or miscarriage:

- Make sure eggs are thoroughly cooked until the whites and yolks are solid.
- Avoid foods containing raw and undercooked eggs like homemade mayonnaise, ice-cream, cheesecake or mousse.

To avoid listeria infection which can lead to miscarriage, stillbirth or severe illness in the newborn:

- Avoid eating all types of paté, including vegetable patés.
- Avoid all unpasteurised milk (or boil it before consumption).
- Avoid all cheese made with unpasteurised milk and mould-ripened soft cheese.

To avoid campylobacter infection which can cause premature labour, still births or spontaneous abortion:

- Avoid raw meat and poultry.
- Untreated surface water.

For general hygiene:

- Wash your hands before and after handling any food especially raw food and after handling soil (e.g. after gardening).
- Store raw food separate from cooked food.

Table 5.11 How much caffeine is there in foods? (British Nutrition Foundation 2004)

- 1 mug of instant coffee contains 100mg caffeine

- 1 cup of brewed coffee contains 100mg caffeine

- 1 can of 'energy' drink contains up to 80mg caffeine

- 1 cup of instant coffee contains 75mg caffeine

- 1 cup of tea contains 50mg caffeine

- 1 chocolate bar (50g) contains up to 50mg caffeine

- 1 can of cola contains up to 40mg caffeine

Conclusion

Unnecessary gestational weight gain and maternal overweight/obesity are associated with some adverse infant and maternal outcomes. A standard weight gain recommendation for all women is not reasonable. To understand fully the impact of gestational weight gain on short and long-term outcomes for women and their offspring, more research with longer follow-up is needed. Current research, however, indicates that for some women, general healthy eating advice may not be sufficient to prevent unnecessary weight gain during pregnancy. For these women, more detailed advice regarding portion control and exercise should be given by health care professionals such as midwives and dietitians. However, pregnant women should adhere to general healthy eating, recommended vitamin and mineral intake, food safety and hygiene guidelines and alcohol and caffeine intake alongside this advice. Unfortunately we do not know how adhering to UK recommendations affects pregnancy weight gain and long term studies are urgently needed.

References

Abrams B, Altman SL, Pickett KE (2000) Pregnancy weight gain: still controversial. *Am J Clin Nutr* **71**(5):1233S-1241S.

American Dietetic Association's Nutrition Care Manual. Normal Pregnancy. http://www.nutritioncaremanual.org (September 2009)

American Dietetic Association (2008) Position of the American Dietetic Association. Nutrition and lifestyle for a healthy pregnancy outcome. *J Am Diet Assoc* **108**: 553–61.

Asbee SM, Jenkins TR, Butler JR *et al* (2009) Preventing excessive weight gain during pregnancy through dietary and lifestyle counseling: a randomized controlled trial. *Obstet Gynecol* **113** (2): 305–312.

British Nutrition Foundation. Maternal and infant nutrition http://www.nutrition.org.uk/home.asp?siteId=43&sectionId=394&subSectionId=315&parentSection=299&which=1 . 2004.

Bruce L, Tchabo JG (1989) Nutrition intervention program in a prenatal clinic. *Obstet Gynecol* **74**(3): 310–12.

Cedergren M (2006) Effects of gestational weight gain and body mass index on obstetric outcome in Sweden. *Int J Gynaecol Obstet* **93**(3): 269-74.

Cetin I, Koletzko B (2008) Long-chain omega-3 fatty acid supply in pregnancy and lactation. *Curr Opin Clin Nutr Metab Care* **11**(3): 297–302.

Claesson IM, Sydsjo G, Brynhildsen J *et al* (2008) Weight gain restriction for obese pregnant women: a case-control intervention study. *BJOG* **115**(1): 44–50.

Committee on Toxicity of Chemicals in Food CpatE. Revised UK Government advice on peanut consumption during early life and allergy risk (2009). http://cot.food.gov.uk/cotstatements/cotstatementsyrs/cotstatements2008/cot200807peanut

Cross Government Obesity Unit. Department of Health (DH) and Department for Children, S. a. F. (2008) *Healthy Weight, Healthy Lives*: *A cross-government strategy for England*. COI, London.

Department of Health (DH) (1991) *Dietary Reference Values for Food Energy and Nutrients in the UK*. *Report on Health and Social Subjects*. HMSO, London: 41.

Department of Health (DH). Definitions of overweight and obesity. http://www.dh.gov.uk/en/Publichealth/Healthimprovement/Obesity/DH_4133948 (September 2009)

DeVader SR, Neeley HL, Myles TD *et al* (2007) Evaluation of gestational weight gain guidelines for women with normal prepregnancy body mass index. *Obstet Gynecol* **110**(4): 745–51.

Dunstan JA, Mori TA, Barden A *et al* (2003) Fish oil supplementation in pregnancy modifies neonatal allergen-specific immune responses and clinical outcomes in infants at high risk of atopy: a randomized, controlled trial. *J Allergy Clin Immunol.* **112**(6): 1178–84.

Feig DS and Naylor CD (1998) Eating for two: are guidelines for weight gain during pregnancy too liberal? *Lancet* **351**(9108): 1054–5.

Food Standards Agency. Eating while you are pregnant. www.eatwell.gov.uk/pregnancy . 2009a.

Food Standards Agency. Folic Acid Fortification. http://www.eatwell.gov.uk/ healthissues/factsbehindissues/folicacid/?lang=en . 2009b.

Frederick et al 2008: Frederick, I. O., Williams, M. A., Sales, A. E., Martin, D. P., & Killien, M. 2008, "Pre-pregnancy body mass index, gestational weight gain, and other maternal characteristics in relation to infant birth weight", Matern. Child Health J, vol. 12 no. 5: 557-67.

Gibson EL (2006) Emotional influences on food choice: sensory, physiological and psychological pathways. *Physiol Behav.* **89**(1): 53–61.

Goldberg G (2003) Nutrition in Pregnancy: The Facts and Fallacies. *Nursing Standard* **17**: 39-42.

Haeri S, Guichard I, Baker AM *et al* (2009) The effect of teenage maternal obesity on perinatal outcomes. *Obstet Gynecol* **113**(2): 300–4.

Haste FM, Brooke OG, Anderson HR *et al* (1990) Nutrient intakes during pregnancy: observations on the influence of smoking and social class. *Am J Clin Nutr* **51**(1): 29–36.

Henderson L, Irving K, Gregory J, *et al* 20093, *National Diet and Nutrition Survey: Adults aged 19 - 64 years. Volume 3: Vitamin and Mineral intake and Urinary analytes.* The Stationery Office, London.

Herring SJ, Oken E, Haines J *et al* (2008) Misperceived prepregnancy body weight status predicts excessive gestational weight gain: findings from a US cohort study. *BMC.Pregnancy Childbirth* **8**: 54.

Heslehurst N, Simpson H, Ells LJ *et al* (2008) The impact of maternal BMI status on pregnancy outcomes with immediate short-term obstetric resource implications: a meta-analysis. *Obes Rev* **9**(6): 635–83.

Heslehurst N, Ells LJ, Simpson H *et al* (2007a) Trends in maternal obesity incidence rates, demographic predictors, and health inequalities in 36,821 women over a 15-year period. *BJOG* **114**(2): 187–94.

Heslehurst N, Lang R, Rankin J *et al* (2007b) Obesity in pregnancy: a study of the impact of maternal obesity on NHS maternity services. *BJOG* **114**(3): 334–2.

Institute of Medicine (IOM) (1990) *Nutrition During Pregnancy*. National Academies Press, Washington DC.

Institute of Medicine. Weight Gain During Pregnancy: Reexamining the Guidelines. http://www.iom.edu/Object.File/Master/68/230/Report%20Brief%20-%20Weight%20Gain%20During%20Pregnancy.pdf . 2009.

Kiel DW, Dodson, EA, Artal R *et al* (2007) Gestational weight gain and pregnancy outcomes in obese women: how much is enough? *Obstet Gynecol* **110**(4): 752–8.

Kinnunen TI, Pasanen M, Aittasalo M *et al* (2007) Preventing excessive weight gain during pregnancy - a controlled trial in primary health care. *Eur J Clin Nutr* **61**(7): 884–91.

National Health Services:

http://www.nhs.uk/livewell/pregnancy/pages/healthyeating.aspx (September 2009)

NICE. National Institute for Health and Clinical Excellence guidelines (2008) *Improving the nutrition of pregnant and breastfeeding mothers and children in low-income households*. London: 105

Olson CM (2008) Achieving a healthy weight gain during pregnancy. *Annu Rev Nutr* **28**: 411–23.

Olson CM, Strawderman MS, Dennison BA (2008) Maternal Weight Gain During Pregnancy and Child Weight at Age 3 Years. *Matern Child Health J*

Olson CM, Strawderman MS, Reed RG (2004) Efficacy of an intervention to prevent excessive gestational weight gain. *Am J Obstet Gynecol* **191**(2): 530–6.

Olson CM, Strawderman MS, Dennison BA (2009) Maternal Weight Gain During Pregnancy and Child Weight at Age 3 Years. Matern Child Health J 13: 839-46

Orstead C, Arrington D, Kamath SK *et al* (1985) Efficacy of prenatal nutrition counseling: weight gain, infant birth weight, and cost-effectiveness. *J Am Diet Assoc* **85**(1): 40–5.

Peacey V, Steptoe A, Sanderman R *et al* (2006) Ten-year changes in sun protection behaviors and beliefs of young adults in 13 European countries. *Prev Med* **43**(6): 460–5.

Polley BA, Wing RR, Sims CJ (2002) Randomized controlled trial to prevent excessive weight gain in pregnant women. *Int J Obes Relat Metab Disord* **26**(11): 1494–502.

Rees JM, Engelbert-Fenton KA, Gong EJ *et al* (1992) Weight gain in adolescents during pregnancy: rate related to birth-weight outcome. *Am J Clin Nutr* **56**(5): 868–73.

Rode L, Hegaard HK, Kjaergaard H *et al* (2007) Association between maternal weight gain and birth weight. *Obstet Gynecol* **109**(6): 1309–15.

Schieve LA, Cogswell ME, Scanlon KS (1998) Trends in pregnancy weight gain within and outside ranges recommended by the Institute of Medicine in a WIC population. *Matern Child Health J* **2**(2): 111–6.

Scottish Nutrition and Dietetic Research Institue (SNDRi). Controlling your portions. *http://www.gcal.ac.uk/sndri/all_health_resources.html#DOMUK* (2005a).

Scottish Nutrition and Dietetic Research Institue (SNDRi). Patient assessment form. *http://www.gcal.ac.uk/sndri/all_health_resources.html#DOMUK* (2005b).

Stotland NE, Cheng YW, Hopkins LM *et al* (2006) Gestational weight gain and adverse neonatal outcome among term infants. *Obstet Gynecol* **108**(3): 635–43.

Strychar IM, Chabot C, Champagne FP *et al* (2000) Psychosocial and lifestyle factors associated with insufficient and excessive maternal weight gain during pregnancy. *J Am Diet Assoc* **100**(3): 353–6.

The Associate Parliamentary Food and Health Forum. Diet and Behaviour. *www.fhf.org.uk/inquiry* (2007).

Thomas B and Bishop J (2007) Body Mass Index. In: Thomas B and Bishop J eds *Manual of Dietetic Practice*. 4th edn Blackwell Publishing Ltd, Oxford: 853.

Thomas B and Bishop J (2007a) Assessment of Nutritional Status. In: Thomas B and Bishop J eds *Manual of Dietetic Practice*. 4th edn Blackwell Publishing Ltd Oxford: 59–70.

Thomas B and Bishop J (2007b) Pregnancy In: Thomas B and Bishop J eds *Manual of Dietetic Practice*. 4th edn, Blackwell Publishing Ltd, Oxford: 256–66.

Thorsdottir I, Torfadottir JE, Birgisdottir BE *et al* (2002) Weight gain in women of normal weight before pregnancy: complications in pregnancy or delivery and birth outcome. *Obstet Gynecol* **99**(5): 799–806.

Walker LO (2007) Managing excessive weight gain during pregnancy and the postpartum period. *J Obstet Gynecol.Neonatal Nurs* **36**(5): 490–500.

Williamson DF, Madans J, Pamuk E (1994) A prospective study of childbearing and 10-year weight gain in US white women 25 to 45 years of age. *Int J Obes Relat Metab Disord* **18**(8): 561–9.

Wolff S, Legarth J, VangSF *et al* (2008) A randomized trial of the effects of dietary counseling on gestational weight gain and glucose metabolism in obese pregnant women. *Int J Obes (Lond)* **32**(3): 495–501.

WrightT and Meyer R (2009) Milk and eggs. In: Skypala I and Venter C eds. *Food Hypersensitvity: Diagnosing and Managing Food Allergies and Intolerance*, Blackwell Ltd. Oxford:117–35.

Useful resources

BMI charts can be obtained from: http://shop.healthforallchildren.co.uk

Sources of nutrition information for pregnancy in the UK -
Patient UK:
http://www.patient.co.uk/showdoc/27000508/

Department of Health - The pregnancy book:
http://www.dh.gov.uk/en/Publicationsandstatistics/Publications/
    PublicationsPolicyAndGuidance/DH_074920

Food Standards Agency:
http://www.eatwell.gov.uk/agesandstages/pregnancy/whenyrpregnant/

British nutrition foundation:
http://www.nutrition.org.uk/home.asp?siteId=43&sectionId=394&subSectionId=31
    5&parentSection=299&which=1 (accessed April 2009)

Chapter 6

Common Medical Problems in Pregnancy Associated with Obesity

Daghni Rajasingam and Hannah Rickard

Introduction

Pregnancy is a joyous time for a mother and her family, and the normal physiological changes her body experiences usually pass uneventfully. Antenatal care can involve minimal, if any, intervention from doctors. However medical problems can occur in pregnancy and occasionally underlying conditions are exacerbated. Some are specific to pregnancy and develop de novo, such as obstetric choestasis or pre clampsia (PE), but other medical conditions are underlying and may be either diagnosed or undiagnosed. One of the roles of the obstetrician and midwife is to identify women at risk of medical problems, to manage those conditions and ensure a safe and satisfying outcome for both mother and baby.

Obesity is one of the most common and most frequently overlooked risk factors for medical problems in pregnancy. Identification and accurate calculation of body mass index (BMI) is vital as advice and care can be given from before conception through to the post-natal period in order to reduce risk and achieve the best possible outcome.

Obese women are more likely to have underlying medical conditions or co-morbidities at the time of conception, such as hypertension, diabetes and vascular and heart disease, which are all affected by pregnancy. They are also more at risk of some conditions specific to pregnancy. These medical problems can be fatal, and obesity is a significant risk factor for maternal mortality. The UK Confidential Inquiry into Maternal and Child Health (CEMACH 2003-05) (Lewis 2007) found that 52% of the women who died from direct or indirect causes were overweight or obese, and 27% had a BMI of 30 or more. In the general, non pregnant population, obesity contributes to more than 30000 deaths per annum in the UK (6% of all deaths) (National Audit Office 2001). In the USA, obesity contributes to 280 000 deaths (Allison et al 1999).

Overall, the National Audit Office (2001) found that it reduces average life expectancy by approximately nine years in the UK population.

In non pregnant populations, obesity has reached epidemic proportions globally and associated medical problems are beginning to put increasing burden on world health services. The same burden exists for maternity services as obese women tend to need more care and resources. Heselhurst et al (2007) studying maternity services in the North-East of England found that care providers felt obesity had a major impact on service provision in terms of increased antenatal visits, equipment and length of hospital stay.

Data is starting to show that globally, young women of reproductive age are getting fatter; the Health Survey for England (Department of Health [DH] 2005) reported that in the UK in 2003, 16% of females aged 16–34 were obese and it is predicted that by 2010 this will have risen to 22%. In the UK, extreme obesity is now proving to be an even greater problem, with one in every 1000 women having a BMI >50 (Knight 2009). In the USA, 61.6% of women aged over 20 are overweight or obese, and these figures are continuing to rise (Healy et al 2004). There are also important racial differences in the incidence of obesity in women, the highest levels consistently being seen in non-white populations, notably Afro-Caribbeans in both the UK and USA (Healey et al 2004; Sebire et al 2001).

These changes are also being seen in pregnant populations and the mean weight at first antenatal visit has also increased by 20% in the past 20 years in the USA (Lu et al 2001). A Scottish study by Kanagalingam (2005) showed that BMI at the first antenatal visit increased by 1.37 kg/m^2 over a 12-year period and also that the proportion of women classified as obese (BMI > 30 kg/m^2) had more than doubled from 9.4% to 18.9% in the same time period. Another English study has shown that the proportion of women who are obese at the start of pregnancy has increased over time from 9.9% in 1990 to 16.0% in 2004 (Heselhurst et al 2004). The same study also found that incidence of obesity reflects socioeconomic status with increasing numbers of obese women were more likely to live in areas with the highest deprivation.

In all, obesity is rising exponentially, especially in young women of childbearing age. Many women are unaware of the increased risk that this places on their body and unborn child. This chapter explores the pathogenesis and management of common maternal medical problems associated with obesity, including those occurring prepregnancy and some diseases specific to pregnancy.

Diabetes Mellitus in pregnancy

Diabetes mellitus (DM) is the most common pre-existing medical problem seen in pregnant women. In the United States, 21 million people (7% of the population) have some form of diagnosed diabetes and another 6 million people may be undiagnosed (Baptiste-Roberts et al 2009). Levels are increasing worldwide as a result of the increasing numbers of obese women and also because of increasing immigration and ethnic diversity. Diabetes occurs in some form in 3-10% of pregnancies but as more young women (and even children) are developing Type 2 diabetes, this is translating to increasing numbers of women of childbearing age suffering from the disease.

Diabetes is characterised by abnormal glucose homeostasis. It is generally classified into Type 1 or Type 2 diabetes, which is present before pregnancy and accounts for about 8% of all cases, or gestational diabetes, which develops during pregnancy and accounts for 92% of diabetes cases (El-Sayad and Lyell 2001). It is not uncommon for women to be newly diagnosed with underlying diabetes for the first time when she is pregnant, as for some women this is the only time they have contact with healthcare professionals. Type 1 Diabetes Mellitus (T1DM) is more common in women of child bearing age, and in the UK accounts for 73% of prepregnancy diabetes (CEMACH 2007). However within certain urban areas the rates of Type 2 Diabetes Mellitus (T2DM) are higher than those of T1DM, probably due to high levels of obesity and ethnic minorities. A study from St Thomas' Hospital in inner London found the overall prevalence of pre-existing diabetes was 0.81% compared to general London prevalence of 0.39%, with 56% of these being T2DM (Watson 2007).

Type I diabetes

Type 1 diabetes is the result of autoimmune destruction of B-cells in the pancreatic Islets. It usually presents in childhood, and results in hyperglycaemia due to an absolute insulin deficiency. It is treated with daily injected insulin and regular blood sugar monitoring. As it is not generally associated with obesity, further discussion of its management is outside the remit of this chapter, but in pregnant patients where Type 1 diabetes and obesity present their pregnancy should be regarded as higher risk.

Type 2 diabetes

Type 2 diabetes is characterised by high blood glucose in the context of insulin resistance and relative insulin deficiency. Older, multiparous, overweight or obese women, and those with a family history are more at risk (CEMACH 2007). Kumari et al (2001) found that in obese patients the risk of pre-existing diabetes mellitus was 10.8 times higher than in normal-weight controls. Racial origin is also a risk factor and diabetes is more common in women of Hispanic, Afro-Caribbean or Asian ethnicity (CEMACH 2007). South Asians have two to four fold higher rates of Type 2 diabetes, develop it on average 10 years earlier, and have more cardiovascular disease than their European counterparts. Although Afro-Caribbeans in the UK also share this higher prevalence of type 2 diabetes, they tend to have more favourable lipid profiles and thus a lower prevalence of cardiovascular disease. Although it has traditionally been defined as a disease of adults, increasing numbers of children, many of whom are obese, are being diagnosed with Type 2 diabetes. This will impact on younger pregnant women. The problem of undiagnosed type 2 diabetes is intimately correlated with the global obesity epidemic. It is equally true that obesity is more common in women from socio-economically deprived areas, thereby compounding the problem of undiagnosed Type 2 diabetes and obesity and deprivation.

Gestational diabetes mellitus (GDM)

Gestational diabetes mellitus (GDM) is defined as 'carbohydrate intolerance of variable severity with onset or first recognition during the present pregnancy' (National Diabetes Data Group 1979). Its prevalence in developed countries has risen from 2.9% to 8.8% over the past two decades (CEMACH 2007), albeit variably, depending on the level of glucose intolerance used to define the condition and the ethnicity and demographics of the population, as GDM is also more common in ethnic populations. In the UK, the prevalence of GDM is increased threefold in the Afro-Caribbean population, six fold in the Arab/Mediterranean population, eight fold in the South-East Asian population, and 11-fold in women from the Indian subcontinent. The definition also covers the small proportion (0.1%) of women diagnosed with underlying diabetes for the first time in pregnancy.

Mothers with pre-existing diabetes are more at risk of first trimester miscarriage and of fetal developmental defects such as cardiac structural abnormalities and cleft palate. All forms of diabetes carry a strong association with both fetal and maternal morbidity. Diabetic mothers are more likely to go into spontaneous preterm labour, develop PE, and have a caesarean section or perineal trauma (CEMACH 2007). Their babies have a higher risk of developing macrosomia, polyhydramnios or polycythaemia, be born prematurely or stillborn, be distressed in labour, have a birth injury, and have postnatal hypoglycaemia (CEMACH 2007).

Pathophysiology of GDM

During pregnancy, a mother's metabolism adjusts to ensure a constant supply of glucose for the growing fetus and the mother. Placental steroid and peptide hormones (e.g., estrogens, progesterone, and human placental lactogen) cause increasing tissue insulin resistance. Hormone levels tend to rise throughout the second and third trimesters causing an increased demand for insulin, especially after meals. Chronic obesity contributes to the increased insulin resistance, most likely because adipose tissue (especially that in the abdomen around internal organs) secretes the hormones and cytokines which increase insulin resistance (*Figure 6.2*). Mean insulin secretion can be up to 50% higher in the third trimester compared to the non pregnant state.

If the mother's pancreas cannot produce enough insulin, maternal and fetal hyperglycemia ensues manifesting as recurrent post-prandial hyperglycemia, and this is the mainstay of the diagnosis of GDM. Raised maternal and fetal glucose levels are accompanied by episodic fetal hyperinsulinaemia which promotes excess nutrient storage and increases secretion of growth hormone, resulting in macrosomia. This postprandial hyperglycaemia also contributes to the accelerated growth exhibited by the fetus.

The energy the fetus uses to convert excess glucose into fat uses valuable oxygen, and this can lead to depletion in fetal oxygen levels. This causes surges in fetal adrenal catecholamines, which, in turn, cause hypertension, cardiac remodelling and hypertrophy, stimulation of erythropoietin, red cell hyperplasia, and increased haematocrit. Polycythaemia occurs in 5-10% of newborns of diabetic mothers and appears to be related to the tightness of glycaemic control. High haematocrit values in the neonate can lead to poor circulation and postnatal jaundice. The intrauterine environment and the way a baby grows are also thought to impact growth and development and health in later life (Barker Hypothesis 1997). Poor growth and a low birth weight has been found to correlate with increased levels of disease in adult life, including hypertension, heart disease, and diabetes.

Screening for GDM

There is no international consensus on when, how and whom to screen for GDM. National UK guidance suggests that all women should be offered a random blood glucose test at some time during their pregnancy. Many units screen using this and an Oral Glucose Tolerance Test (OGTT), based on clinical risk factors such as previous GDM, family history, obesity, ethnicity, previous macrosomic baby, glycosuria, polyhydramnios, maternal age, and previous stillbirth. Some units advocate universal screening depending on the prevalence of GDM in the local population. It is important to be aware of the possibility of undiagnosed T2DM.

Women should be identified as being at risk of developing GDM and should be referred early antenatally and seen by a dedicated multi-disciplinary team. Risk factors for GDM include;

- Obesity (BMI above 30 kg/m2)
- Previous macrosomic baby weighing 4.5 kg or above.
- Previous gestational diabetes.
- First-degree relative with diabetes.
- Family origin with a high prevalence of diabetes (South Asian, black Caribbean and Middle Eastern).

According to UK National Institute for Health and Clinical Excellence (NICE 2008), if a woman has one or more of these risk factors, a glucose tolerance test (GTT) should be performed at 24-28 weeks. If the woman has had previous GDM or there are suspicions she might have T2DM, glucose monitoring should be undertaken, and this should be brought forward to 16–18 weeks, followed by OGTT at 28 weeks if the first test is normal. The optimal timing for screening also lacks international consensus. Higher detection rates will obviously occur later in pregnancy as mother's insulin resistance increases, but later screening clearly misses the opportunity to treat hyperglycaemia early and thereby improve maternal and fetal outcomes.

The World Health Organisation (WHO) and the UK's NICE (2008) guidelines, diagnostic criteria for diabetes mellitus are as follows, and requires one of the following conditions to be met;

- Fasting plasma glucose >7.0 mmol/L OR
- Plasma glucose of >7.8 mmol/L, two hour following a 75mg oral glucose tolerance test (OGTT).

The American Diabetes Association (2004) has slightly different cut-off levels of fasting plasma blood glucose of >5.3mm/L (>95mg/dL) and 2 hours post 100g oral GTT of >8.6mm/L (>155g/dL). Local policies should always be referred to when screening for diabetes. The classic symptoms of diabetes include polyuria, polydipsia, and unexplained weight loss, but often women are asymptomatic.

Pre-existing diabetes mellitus is higher in women with obesity, and the incidence of gestational diabetes increases proportionally to the BMI, so it is essential that all obese women should be screened during their pregnancy. A meta-analysis of studies of obesity found that the unadjusted odds ratios (ORs) of developing GDM were 2.14 (95% CI 1.82–2.53), 3.56 (3.05– 4.21), and 8.56 (5.07–16.04) among overweight, obese, and severely obese compared with normal-weight pregnant women, respectively (Chu et al 2007). In morbidly obese women, the incidence of GDM is as high as 24.5% (OR 22.6) (Kumari 2001).

Management

All women with prepregnancy diabetes should be seen, and ideally referred to see an obstetrician and/or endocrinologist, for prepregnancy counselling regarding diet, weight management, glycaemic control and potential complications. They should also be advised to take high dose (5mg) folic acid daily to reduce risks of congenital anomaly. The UK CEMACH (2007) Diabetes Programme found that women with diabetes are generally very poorly prepared for pregnancy, with less than half having any counselling, and two-thirds had evidence of suboptimal glycaemic control pre-conception.

Women with T2DM should have targets set for glycaemic monitoring and control in pregnancy and most are treated with insulin to establish this. Retinal and renal screening should be performed along with regular fetal ultrasounds and antenatal visits and a structured plan for delivery should be made (CEMACH 2007).

The exact management of gestational diabetic mothers has been much debated and researched but it is clear that intensive treatment and monitoring, and tight glycaemic control is beneficial. The 2005 ACHOIS trial randomized 1000 women with mild GDM to routine antenatal care or intensive monitoring and blood glucose optimization and found the group managed with intensive interventions such as dietary advice, glucose monitoring, and insulin therapy had significantly improved perinatal outcomes without an increase in rates of caesarean section (Crowther 2005). The National Institute for Health and Clinical Excellence (2008) recommends that women with diabetes should aim to keep fasting blood glucose between 3.5 and 5.9 mmol/litre and one hour postprandial blood glucose below 7.8 mmol/l during pregnancy. The large Hyperglycaemia and Adverse Pregnancy Outcomes HAPO study (2008) also found that women with GDM were at increased risk of having a large baby, needing a cesarean delivery, clinical neonatal hypoglycemia and high cord c-peptide (related to fetal insulin levels) in the newborn. They also found that women who were just below the diagnostic criteria for GDM still carried an increased risk of adverse outcomes and the higher the blood glucose level, the higher the risk. It may be that in the future, diagnostic criteria will be more stringent.

Treatment involves trying to maintain normoglycaemia and increase insulin sensitivity by decreasing fat stores. Obese women should be advised to increase daily exercise, maintain a stable weight through pregnancy, and adopt a low-calorie, low-fat diet. They should eliminate sugary drinks, and increase fibre and complex carbohydrate consumption. If blood glucose levels remain elevated despite dietary changes, patients should be started on antiglycaemics. In obese women, even with optimal glycaemic control on diet alone, adverse pregnancy outcomes such as metabolic complications, macrosomia or neontal intensive care unit (NICU) admissions are still two to three fold higher in obese patients treated with insulin, suggesting there should be a low threshold for treatment. The first-line treatment is usually subcutaneous insulin, and the exact regimen depends on local guidelines.

Traditionally, oral hypoglycaemic agents were not recommended, however data from retrospective trials of women treated with metformin for polycystic ovarian syndrome (PCOS) who continued taking it during part, or all of their pregnancy, show that it is safe in pregnancy without increased risk of neonatal hypoglycaemia, fetal anomalies, or malformations (Homko and Reece 2006; Ho et al 2007). The recently published 2009 Metformin in Gestational Diabetes (MiG) study comparing insulin with metformin has also shown that it is safe and reduces insulin resistance, and has comparable neonatal outcomes to insulin (Rowan 2008). Some 46% of women also needed supplementary insulin to maintain sugar control but metformin reduced insulin requirement. First generation sulphonylureas has been avoided in pregnancy because of the potential risk of teratogenicity and neonatal hypoglycemia, but increasingly in the US and UK, glibenclamide (glyburide) is being prescribed. It has minimal placental transfer and in a randomised controlled trial of glibenclamide versus insulin in gestational diabetes, Langer et al (2000) showed there were no significant differences in perinatal or neonatal outcomes or maternal glycaemic control between both the groups and only 4% of patients needed extra insulin therapy.

This new evidence in favour of oral agents may be of particular relevance to the developing world, where rates of obesity and diabetes in pregnancy are increasing. The cultural beliefs may be at odds with the use of insulin injections. The cost and practicalities of storing insulin may also limit its use.

Postnatally, women with GDM usually stop their medication immediately as glucose homeostasis returns to normal quickly. Women with GDM should be counselled about their increased risk of diabetes in future pregnancies and should also be given dietary and exercise advice with the aim of losing weight and reducing their risk of Type 2 diabetes and cardiovascular disease in later life. Women who develop GDM are at increased risk of type 2 diabetes in the long term, with 40% developing it in the future (Bachanan and Kjos 1999). There needs to be good communication with the general practitioner who should organise a repeat glucose tolerance test (GTT) six weeks postnatally to establish whether underlying type 2 diabetes is present.

Hypertension

In normal pregnancy, blood pressure falls in early to mid pregnancy as a result of progesterone induced vasodilatation. It continues to decrease in the second trimester until about 22–24 weeks gestation, then rises steadily to prepregnancy values at term, mainly due to increased cardiac output by 30-50%, and blood volume up to 50%.

Hypertension is one of the most common medical problems in pregnancy, occurring in some form in 10–15% of all pregnancies. There is a spectrum of hypertensive disorders, from mild essential hypertension, to full-blown eclampsia. Worldwide, hypertension is a leading cause of maternal morbidity and mortality. In South Africa, for example, complications of hypertension in pregnancy are the most common direct cause of death and the second most common cause of all maternal deaths (15.7%) after HIV (South Africa DH 2004). In the UK, the CEMACH 2003–2005 report listed 14 deaths over the three year period related to hypertensive complications (Lewis 2007). Obesity is a risk factor for all forms of hypertensive disease in pregnancy, and obese mothers should be informed of this in early pregnancy and referred for obstetrician led care according to the Pre-clampsia Community Guidelines (PRECOG) (Action on PE 2004) .

Monitoring of blood pressure also represents an additional problem in obese women, as blood pressure can be overestimated if a small sphygmomanometer cuff is used, and this can lead to wrong diagnosis or inappropriate treatment. A correctly sized cuff should be used – usually standard size for an arm circumference of up to 33 cm, a large size for an arm circumference 33-41 cm and a thigh cuff for an arm circumference of >41 cm (Action on PE 2004). There is less error introduced by using too large a cuff than by too small a cuff. The Korotkoff V sound (disappearance of the heart sounds) should be taken as the diastolic reading, as this is reproducible and better related to outcome.

Pre-existing hypertension

Pre-existing (essential) hypertension in the general adult population is a major risk factor for cardio- and cerebrovascular disease such as haemorrhagic stroke, ischaemic heart disease and peripheral vascular disease. It is defined as a systolic blood pressure of 140 mmHg or greater, and/or a diastolic blood pressure of 90 mmHg or more, either prepregnancy or at an early antenatal visit (before 12 weeks gestation). It can occur in all age groups and affects 1–5% of pregnant women (National High Blood Pressure Working Group 1990). It is a risk factor for PE, placental abruption, and fetal compromise.

The incidence of pre-existing hypertension in pregnancy increases with age and is multifactorial in aetiology. Common risk factors are genetics, race, and diet, but in obese women, the incidence of pre-existing hypertension increases to 4.3% (Kumari 2001).

Management

In any young woman presenting with hypertension, a secondary cause must be considered prior to initiating treatment and a full assessment with physical examination and investigations including renal profile and electrocardiogram (ECG).

If diet and weight loss fails, medical treatment should be considered. The main aim of control should be systolic blood pressure as this is the greatest risk factor for haemorrhagic stroke. Appropriate medication recognized to be safe in pregnancy should be used, based on national guidelines. Any woman with known pre-existing hypertension, already taking antihypertensive medication should be advised to switch to a recommended drug regime during the pregnancy and when breastfeeding. Even with medication, blood pressure may increase as the pregnancy progresses and women with essential hypertension are at increased risk of developing one of the two pregnancy hypertensive disorders – pregnancy induced hypertension or PE. Essential hypertension is also a risk factor for other comorbidites, and health providers should be aware of the potential of ischaemic heart disease (IHD), or cerebrovascular disease, especially in mothers over the age of 35. The UK CEMACH report, cardiac disease was the commonest cause of maternal death overall, and 33% of these were due to IHD (Lewis 2007).

Pregnancy-Induced Hypertension (PIH)

This disorder, specific to pregnancy, is defined as hypertension developing after 20 weeks' gestation and resolving within six weeks of delivery. It affects 5–10% of pregnancies and is more common in primigravid women (25% incidence). It is not normally serious, but with increasing maternal weight and obesity, this risk increases greatly (Weiss et al 2004, Bodnar et al 2007). Although the exact cause of PIH is unknown, it seems to be part of a spectrum of pregnancy disorders ranging from PE, HELLP (haemolysis elevated liver enzymes and low platelets) syndrome and haemolytic uraemic syndrome (Freidman 2006). The pathology may be the result of abnormal placental invasion and immune mediated reaction and inflammation.

Management

Antenatal care should include a record of blood pressure at the initial and every subsequent antenatal visit. It is important to monitor patients for emerging PE with urinalysis and blood tests. Antihypertensive medication is not always indicated, but moderate and severe hypertension does require treatment and persistent monitoring. Treatment is recommended if the systolic pressure exceeds 160 mmHg or the diastolic exceeds 110 mmHg. In the UK, methyldopa is usually the first-line antihypertensive used in pregnancy but labetalol, nifedipine SR, and hydralazine are also safe. Angiotensin-converting enzyme (ACE) inhibitors and angiotensin receptor antagonists should be avoided in the first trimester, as they have been associated with congenital abnormalities and fetal death.

Pregnancy induced hypertension may also be a precursor for PE, so regular urinalysis for proteinurea and blood monitoring of renal and liver function and platelet count should performed to check for the development of this.

Pre eclampsia (PE)

Pre eclampsia is a multisystem disorder that most commonly occurs in the second half of pregnancy. Classically, it includes the triad of high blood pressure, proteinuria, and oedema, but its manifestations are widespread and often involve the renal, hepatic, neurologic and haematologic systems. It is a generalised disease of the endothelium. Blood vessels develop abnormalities of constriction, affecting blood pressure, and the reflexes become hyperactive. High blood pressure is defined as blood pressure above 140/90 mmHg on two separate occasions four hours apart, or a single diastolic pressure of 110 mmHg. The appearance of hypertension is usually in association with new-onset significant proteinuria on dipstick or quantified proteinuria over 0.3 g/ 24 hours. Some units also use urine protein-creatinine ratio as a more rapid estimation of proteinuria. The kidneys are especially vulnerable in PE, affecting filtration, and resulting in the excretion of protein in the urine and thus generalised peripheral oedema.

Obesity is a well-recognised risk factor for PE, and a large number of international studies from Europe, America, and the Middle East show a clear association between maternal obesity and increasing incidence of hypertensive disorders in pregnancy (Bodnar et al 2007, Bhattacharya et al 2007, Magnussen et al 2007). In all of these studies the incidence and adjusted relative risk of developing PE increase concomitantly with increasing BMI (*Figure 6.1*). In another review of 13 studies, totalling over

1.3 million women, the risk of PE doubled with each 5–7-unit increase in BMI (O'Brien et al 2003). A similar pattern in PE incidence is seen with increasing early pregnancy waist circumference, suggesting it is also a sensitive marker for identifying women at risk of PE (Magnussen et al 2007; Satlar et al 2001). A UK study looking at obese pregnant women found that 11.7% developed PE, with 1.8% diagnosed before 34 weeks' gestation (early-onset PE). The incidence of PE increased with BMI, from 8.3% (BMI 30-34 kg/m2) to 19% (BMI >40 kg/m2) (adjusted OR 2.9; 95% CI, 1.3 to 6.9, P=.010) (Rajasingam 2009).

Other risk factors for PE are numerous, including family history, multiple pregnancy, pre-existing hypertension, increased maternal age, primiparity, and co-existing medical conditions such as renal disese. Ethnic origin is also important; interestingly Bodnar et al (2007) found that obese white women have a higher risk of PE and hypertension than obese Afro-Caribbean women, whereas in normal weight women, this trend is reversed, and white women have a lower risk of hypertensive disorder.

Pathogenesis

The pathogenesis of PE is thought to involve a failure of adequate placentation and an abnormal inflammatory and immune response by the mother to the placenta and the fetus, although the exact mechanism is unknown. Increased

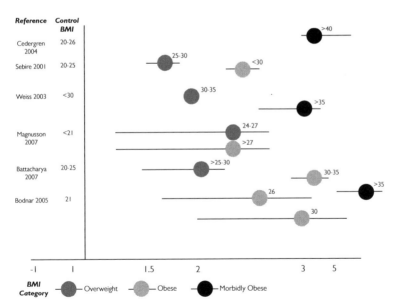

Figure 6.1 Comparison of risk of PE within different weight categories, categorised by BMI.

levels of inflammatory factors and cytokines, including tumour necrosis factor (TNF)-α, interleukin (IL)-1, and IL-6 occur in women with PE. The inflammatory response causes widespread endothelial dysfunction (Roberts 1998; Freeman et al 2004), resulting in proteinuria due to renal glomerular dysfunction, hypertension due to vasoconstriction and generalized peripheral and facial oedema due to increased vascular permeability. The pulmonary circulation is also vulnerable, and women with severe PE are at high risk of developing life-threatening pulmonary oedema.

In obese women, the increased likelihood of developing PE may be due to the mother's altered metabolic state. High body fat levels correlate with increased levels of inflammatory mediators (*Figure 6.2*), and are thought to make such individuals more susceptible to the condition. Adipose tissue also produces proinflammatory cytokines, such as leptin and CRP and triglycerides. Elevated levels of these in early pregnancy correlate with, and are thought to contribute to, increased risk of developing PE later in pregnancy (Bodnar et al 2005; Wolf et al 2001). The increased risk of diabetes and thrombus are also thought to be linked to that of PE, though complex inflammatory interactions are thought to occur as a result of high body fat levels (*Figure 6.2*).

The idea that PE is due to an inflammatory process is given further weight by Sattar et al (1996) who speculate that pregnant women with central abdominal obesity have increased insulin resistance and dyslipidaemia. The

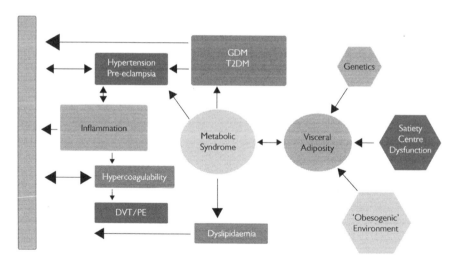

Figure 6.2 The interacting factors that contribute to medical problems in pregnancy for obese women.

associated hyperinsulinaemia leads to increased lipid breakdown in visceral fat, increased concentration of fatty acids in the portal circulation, and thus abnormal synthesis of triglycerides in the liver, and the accumulation of free triglyceride in hepatocytes, leading to liver dysfunction and 'fatty liver'. The increased synthesis of very-low density lipoprotein (VLDL) and low-density lipoprotein (LDL) by the liver contributes to PE, as these particles promote endothelial cell activation and expression of adhesion molecules and decreased levels of high-density lipoprotein (HDL) cholesterol.

Women who have pre-existing cardiovascular risk factors, such as hypertension or high cholesterol, at their first antenatal visit are at increased risk of developing PE. Furthermore, women who suffer from PE are also at increased lifetime risk of hypertension and vascular disease (Bellamy et al 2007). This adds weight to suggestions that PE and all vascular diseases are linked by a common mechanism of chronic inflammation and endothelial dysfunction.

Bodnar et al (2005) have shown that inflammation and increased triglyceride levels account for only about 30% of the effect that prepregnancy BMI has on PE risk. It is still unclear exactly which other factors play the most significant part in the development and progression of the disease.

Severe PE may develop rapidly into eclampsia, characterized by cerebral oedema and seizures. Other life-threatening consequences of the disease include renal and hepatic failure, disseminated intravascular coagulation (DIC), and HELLP syndrome. The fetus may be growth restricted as a result of poor placental function. Eclampsia occurs in approximately 1–2% of women with PE in the developed world, equating to 0.05% of all pregnancies and remains an important cause of maternal mortality globally.

Management

The most important factor in the management of hypertensive disease is regular monitoring in women at risk, for example obese, family history, or multiple pregnancies. In the UK, PRECOG guidelines recommend women with BMI >35 be referred for consultant obstetric care, and be seen for blood pressure checks at no less than two week intervals in the third trimester (APEC 2004). Early recognition and management of women with symptoms and signs of PE, such as headache, visual disturbances, oedema, and liver capsule pain, as well as symptom recognition, should be taught antenatally.

Antihypertensives should be used as for PIH, with especial care to maintain the systolic BP below 160mmHg. No one class of drug is known to be superior in obese women. Women with severe PE may need intravenous medication in the peri-partum period but the only definitive, curative treatment of PE is delivery of the baby and placenta.

The criteria for diagnosis is that new onset hypertension should be seen in addition to new onset significant urine protein excretion (over 0.3 g/24 hours), in the absence of any underlying renal disorder. Quantification of proteinuria is usually done from a sample collected over a 24-hour period but single sample urine protein-creatinine (PCR) is also used as it is much quicker. Patients with underlying renal disease should have their baseline 24-hour protein excretion level checked at the first antenatal visit. Monthly monitoring of full blood count, liver function, renal function, electrolytes, and serum urate is appropriate, but if PE is diagnosed, surveillance should be increased to bi-weekly at least. If thrombocytopenia is present, clotting studies should be performed.

Uterine artery Doppler performed in the second trimester can predict a high risk of developing PE. In obese women with hypertension there may be an increase in intrauterine growth retardation so regular growth scans are important. Fetal well-being should be monitored by repeated ultrasound scanning. Nutritional status of obese women, especially those from deprived areas, is also thought to contribute to poor fetal growth. In a study of obese women living in urban settings, Rajasingam et al (2009) found that there was a high incidence of fetal growth restriction in obese nulliparous women, but interestingly more than 50% was unrelated to developing PE. There may be some as yet unidentified nutritional factors from the diet of obese women that contributes to poor fetal growth.

Antiplatelet agents, such as low dose aspirin, have small to moderate benefit when used early for prevention of PE but only in women with a history of previous early-onset PE. While there are no data for its effect specifically in obese women, the rationale for considering its use exists (Askie et al 2007). Given the supposed role of nutrient deficiency, oxidative stress, and inflammation in PE, a role for antioxidants, especially vitamin C and vitamin E, in its prevention has been suggested. However, in a large, randomized, controlled trial on Vitamins in Pregnancy (VIP), no reduction in PE was found in women with vitamin C and E supplementation and there was actually an increase in the incidence of low birth weight babies. The trial also included a small cohort of obese women in whom vitamin supplementation also was not associated with a decrease in PE (Poston et al 2006).

Venous thromboembolus (VTE)

Venous thromboembolus is another important medical problem that is associated with pregnancy, due to the hypercoagulable pregnant state. Thromboembolic disease is a leading cause of direct maternal death across the world, and is the most common cause of death in the UK. In the UK

CEMACH report of 2003–05, 33 deaths were recorded from pulmonary embolism (PE) and eight from cerebral vein thrombosis (1.56 per 100 000) (Lewis 2007). In Australia, there were two direct deaths from VTE in the 750 000 births from 2000 (Australian Institute of Health and Welfare 2002) . Pre eclampsia has a mortality rate of about 2.5%, so for each fatal PE, there are 40 non-fatal (Knight 2008), and many more DVTs. Of the 33 women who died from PE in the UK in 2003–5, about 50% were overweight or obese (Lewis 2007). The correlation between obesity and risk of PE is evident and must be taken into consideration when caring for women, especially when risk evaluating for thromboprophylaxis.

The overall risk of developing VTE either during or after pregnancy regardless of BMI is about 0.1%, approximately three times the risk in the non pregnant population aged <40. A study from Scotland estimated 0.7 deep vein thrombosis (DVT) and 0.21 pulmonary embolisms (PE) per 1000 deliveries (McColl et al 1997). In obese pregnant women however, the incidence of developing DVT is thought to be much higher but relatively few studies have looked specifically at this, possibly because the numbers of both conditions are small. In a Danish study (Larsen et al 2007) of 126 783 women, obesity in early pregnancy was found to significantly increase the risk of VTE (OR 5.3, CI 2.1, 13.5). In a large study of pregnant women in the UK, the prevalence of PE in overweight women was 0.07% and in obese women 0.08% compared to 0.04% in normal-weight women (Sebire et al 2001). Although clinically important, this difference was not statistically significant. The UK Obstetric Surveillance System Report (UKOSS) 2007 found that BMI over 30 is a major risk factor for PE (OR 2.8, CI 1.12, 7.02) (Knight et al 2007). In the non pregnant population, obesity has also been associated with increased incidence of DVT and the same is probably true in pregnancy (Tsai et al 2002).

Pathogenesis

The maternal coagulation and fibrinolytic systems change dramatically as a physiologic adaptation in preparation for the need for haemostasis following delivery of the baby and placenta. Synthesis of procoagulant factors, such as factors VIII, IX, and X, increases fibrinogen levels by 50%, along with a suppression of fibrinolysis and reduction in antithrombin and protein S levels (Vaya et al 2007). The result is a shift in the balance of the clotting system in favour of a 'hypercoagulable' state in order to prevent haemorrhage at delivery, but for this reason, pregnant and recently delivered women are also at increased risk of venous thrombosis. For a thrombus to arise, the classical Virchow's triad of venous stasis, hypercoagulability, and injury to the intima of veins must be present. Venous flow normally decreases by 50% in all pregnancies, and stasis is exacerbated by prolonged periods of bed rest, immobility after caesarean section, or long-haul travel. The hypercoagulable state can be further increased by many disorders, such as inherited and acquired thrombophilia and underlying malignancy, and anatomical compression of the veins by the gravid uterus. In pregnancy, over 80 % of deep vein thrombosis (DVT) lesions are located on the left side (Ginsburg et al 1992) due to the compression of the left iliac vein by the overlying right iliac and ovarian arteries. Most of these are on the left side due to the compression of the left iliac vein by the overlying right iliac and ovarian arteries. Injury to the vascular endothelium, especially of the pelvic veins, may occur during operative delivery or at the time of caesarean section (CS).

Relatively little is known about the physiologic reasons for the increased risk of VTE in obese mothers. Theories include increased activation of endothelial cells, increased inflammatory mediators, and reduction in antithrombotic agents, such as prostacyclin (PGI2), which is produced by vessel endothelial cells and acts as an inhibitor of platelet aggregation (*Figure 6.2*). Studies have shown that PGI2 levels are reduced in obese patients and in PE pregnancies, and there is speculation that this may contribute to the risk. Another suggested reason for the increase of VTE in obese women is that they tend to have more sedentary lifestyles and are overall less likely to participate in any form of exercise thus continuing to increase venous stasis.

Thromboprophylaxis

Thromboprophylaxis against VTE in the antenatal period should be offered on the basis of the individual women's risk profile. It is not routinely given to all obese women during pregnancy. If a woman has had a previous VTE, is known to have underlying thrombophilia, or has several (usually more than three) persisting risk factors for VTE, of which obesity is one, prophylaxis should be offered (Royal College of Obstetricians and Gynaecologists [RCOG] 2004).

Other risk factors include prolonged bed rest, dehydration, surgery or immobility. Low molecular weight heparin (LMWH) is the most commonly used prophylaxis at a dose of 40 mg enoxaparin once daily (or 500 U dalteparin once daily/4500 U tinzaparin once daily) for normal-weight women in pregnancy and the puerperium. If patients weigh over 90 kg, or have a BMI over 35, it is recommended that this dose be given twice daily (e.g., enoxaparin 40 mg once daily) (RCOG 2004). It is important to educate women that LMWH is safe in pregnancy and breastfeeding as it does not cross the placenta or pass into breast milk.

Postpartum, all women who have had CS should be given LMWH prophylaxis for the duration of their inpatient stay, irrespective of their weight. Obese women (BMI >30) who have had vaginal deliveries should also be offered LMWH for up to 5 days post partum, especially if they have other current risk factors for VTE, such as immobility, PE, prolonged labour, excessive blood loss, or instrumental delivery (RCOG 2004). The postnatal prophylactic dose regimens are the same as those used antenatally and it should be given as soon as possible after delivery, provided there is no postpartum haemorrhage. If an obese woman is discharged home prior to completing her course of LMWH, she should be given the remaining doses to self-administer at home. Good clinical practice should encourage all women to keep well hydrated and to mobilize early. Women who are inpatients should also be advised to wear class I graduated compression stockings while in hospital and for up to six weeks post partum.

Clinical thromboembolism

Clinical features of DVT include leg or groin pain, tenderness, swelling and oedema, overlying skin warmth, and superficial venous dilatation. Venous thromboses sometimes begin in the leg veins, which then extend proximally where they attach to the vein wall, limiting venous return, or they may remain loose in the vessel lumen. This is more dangerous as they often do not have symptoms and are difficult to detect clinically until they embolise to the pulmonary circulation.

Pre eclampsia presents clinically with breathlessness, pleuritic chest pain, cough, and haemoptysis, sometimes in association with leg symptoms but two-thirds of patients with PE do not have any symptoms of DVT. Clinical examination may reveal tachycardia, tachypnoea, and hypoxia, especially on exertion. In cases of severe PE, the patient may present shocked or collapsed, with signs of right heart strain such as jugular vein distension and right ventricular heave. Atypical presentations are common, and a high index of suspicion in pregnancy is required.

Investigation

If a mother's clinical presentation is suspicious enough of VTE to merit investigation, then she should be offered treatment dose low-molecular weight heparin (see below). Treatment should continue until the VTE is excluded using appropriate imaging. It is important that the correct diagnosis is made as there are major implications for this and future pregnancies.

Investigations should include the following:

Venous Doppler scanning
This is normally the first-line investigation. It is sensitive for detection of most above-knee DVT, but its use is limited in very obese patients due to their large body habitus and subcutaneous fat layer.

Venography
If available, this study is preferable in obese patients, but it is an invasive investigation, and involves radiation exposure so it is not ideal in pregnancy.

The diagnosis of PE should involve a full range of tests to exclude other causes of chest pain and breathlessness:

Chest radiography may be normal, but signs to look for include pleural effusion, lobar collapse, or areas of translucency due to hypoperfusion. It is also useful in excluding other causes for respiratory distress such as pneumonia or pneumothorax.

Lung perfusion (Q) or ventilation/perfusion (V/Q) scans. Inhalation of radioactive xenon-133 combined with intravenous radiation identifies areas of mismatched blood flow.

Computerized tomography pulmonary angiogram (CT–PA). This investigation is regarded as safe in pregnancy. The radiation dose to the fetus is minimal, but maternal breast tissue is exposed to moderate radiation.

D-dimers. This is not usually a useful investigation, as it is invariably elevated in all pregnancies, but if negative, this can usually exclude a diagnosis of PE.

Arterial blood gas analysis may reveal hypoxaemia and hypocapnea (due to hyperventilation).

Electrocardiography (ECG) may be normal except for sinus tachycardia. Some patients may have signs of right heart strain, including right-axis deviation, right bundle branch block, and peaked P-waves.

Full blood count (FBC). The white cell and neutrophil count is often raised in patients with PE. It should not be taken as false reassurance that breathlessness is due to infection.

Pulmonary angiography involves the highest radiation exposure and is not normally recommended.

Treatment of VTE

The treatment of confirmed VTE is usually LMWH at a dose which is dependent on the patient's body weight and whether treatment is antenatal or postpartum. During pregnancy, the pharmacokinetic properties of some LMWHs are altered, so a twice-daily dosage regimen is recommended (enoxaparin 1 mg/kg twice daily, dalteparin 100 U/kg twice daily) (RCOG 2008). Treatment should begin prior to any investigations if there is a high clinical index of suspicion. Unstable or collapsed patients should be treated by a multidisciplinary team and intravenous unfractioned heparin is the treatment of choice, but in extreme circumstances, immediate thrombolysis or embolectomy may be considered. An inferior-vena caval filter can be considered in patients presenting with recurrent PE.

When VTE is confirmed, screening for acquired and inherited thrombophilia is required, including protein C, protein S, factor V Leiden, antithrombin deficiency, antiphospholipid antibodies, lupus anticoagulant, and anticardiolipin antibodies. The patient must be treated for three months, including six weeks postnatally. Either LMWH or warfarin can be offered as a long-term thromboprophylaxis postnatally, as both are safe in breastfeeding. Warfarin is usually started on day three postpartum due to the risk of bleeding. LMWH must be continued until an adequate international, normalized ratio (INR) is achieved.

Conclusion

All of the above common medical problems can result in poor pregnancy outcomes for the mother and baby. As the obesity epidemic increases unchecked, we all have a public health responsibility to educate women and their families prepregnancy, in order to impart information to the public about obesity, its effects on pregnancy and about optimising weight and health prior to planning a pregnancy . There needs to be a balance between risk stratifying these women as high risk and yet enabling them to have as normal a pregnancy and delivery as possible.

References

Action on PE (APEC) (2004) *Pre-ecampsia Community Guideline (PRECOG)*. Middlesex: Action on PE.

Allison DB, Fontaine KR, Manson JE, et al (1999) Annual deaths attributable to obesity in the United States. *JAMA* **282**:1530-8.

American Diabetes Association (2004) Gestational diabetes mellitus (Position Statement). *Diabetes Care* 27 (Suppl. 1):S88–S90

Barker DJ (1997)"Maternal Nutrition, Fetal Nutrition, and Disease in Later Life". *Nutrition* **13**:807-13

Askie LM, Duley L, Henderson-Smart DJ, Stewart LA and PARIS Collaborative Group (2007) Antiplatelet agents for prevention of PE: a meta-analysis of individual patient data. *Lancet* **369**:1791–8.

Baptiste-Roberts K, Barone BB, Gary TL, et al (2009) Risk factors for type 2 diabetes among women with gestational diabetes: a systematic review. *Am J Med*. **122**(3):207-214

Bellamy L, Casas J-P, Hingorani AD et al (2007) PE and risk of cardio-vascular disease and cancer in later life: systematic review and metaanalysis. *BMJ* **335**:974–7.

Bhattacharya S, Campbell DM, Liston WA et al (2007) Effect of body mass index on pregnancy outcomes in nulliparous women delivering singleton babies. *BMC Public Health* **7**:168.

Bodnar LM, Catov JM, Klebanoff MA, et al. (2007) Pre-pregnancy body mass index and the occurrence of severe hypertensive disorders of pregnancy. *Epidemiology* **18**:234–9.

Bodnar LM, Ness RB, Harger GF et al (2005) Inflammation and triglycerides partially mediate the effect of prepregnancy body mass index on the risk of PE. *Am J Epidemiol* **162**:1198–206.

Buchanan T, Kjos S. (1999) Gestational Diabetes: risk or myth? *Journal of Clinical Endocrinology and Metabolism* **84**:1854-7.

Cedergren MI. (2004) Maternal morbid obesity and the risk of adverse pregnancy outcome. *Obstet Gynecol* **103**:219–24.

Chu SY, Callaghan WM, Kim SY, et al (2007)Maternal obesity and risk of gestational diabetes mellitus. *Diabetes Care* **30**:2070–6.

Confidential Enquiry into Maternal and Child Health. (2007) Diabetes in Pregnancy: Are we providing the best care? Findings of a National Enquiry: England, Wales and Northern Ireland. CEMACH: London

Crowther CA, Hiller JE, Moss JR, et al (2005) for ACHOIS Collaborative Group. Effect of treatment of mild gestational diabetes mellitus on pregnancy outcomes. The ACHOIS randomized controlled trial. *N Engl J Med* **352**:2477–86.

Department of Health (2005) *Forecasting obesity to 2010*. Health Survey for England. London: DH.

El-Sayed YY and Lyell DJ (2001).New therapies for the pregnant patient with diabetes. *Diabetes Technology and Therapeutics* **3**: 635-40.

Freeman DJ, McManus F, Brown EA, et al.(2004) Short- and long-term changes in plasma inflammatory markers associated with PE. *Hypertension* **43**:708–14.

Friedman JM (2006) ACE inhibitors and congenital anomalies. *N Engl J Med* **354**:2498-500.

Ginsberg JS, Brill-Edwards P, Burrows RF et al (1992). Venous thrombosis during pregnancy: leg and trimester of presentation. *Thromb Haemost*; **67**: 519-20

Hedley AA, Ogden CL, Johnson CL, et al (2004) Prevalence of overweight and obesity among US children, adolescents, and adults, 1999–2002. *JAMA* **291**:2847–50.

Heslehurst N, Laing R, Rankin J, et al.(2007) Obesity in pregnancy: a study of the impact of maternal obesity on NHS maternity services. *BJOG* **114**:334-342

Heslehurst N, Ells L, Simpson H et al (2007) Trends in maternal obesity incidence rates, demographic predictors, and health inequalities in 36 821 women over a 15-year period. *BJOG* **114**:187-194

Ho FL, Liew CF, Cunanan EC, Lee KO. (2007) Oral hypoglycaemic agents for diabetes in pregnancy – an appraisal of the current evidence for oral antidiabetic drug use in pregnancy. *Ann Acad Med Singapore* **36**:672–8.

Homko CJ, Reece EA. (2006) Insulins and oral hypoglycemic agents in pregnancy. *J Matern Fetal Neonatal Med* **19**:679–86.

Kanagalingam MG, Forouhi NG, Greer IA et al (2005) Changes in booking body mass index over a decade: retrospective analysis from a Glasgow Maternity Hospital. *BJOG* **112**:1431–3.

Knight M, Kurinczuk JJ, Spark P, Brocklehurst P. United Kingdom Obstetric Surveillance System (UKOSS) Annual Report 2007. Oxford: National Perinatal Epidemiology Audit.

Knight M on behalf of UKOSS. Antenatal pulmonary embolism: risk factors, management and outcomes. BJOG 2008;115:453–461

Knight M, Kurinczuk JJ, Spark P and Brocklehurst P on behalf of UKOSS. United Kingdom Obstetric Surveillance System (UKOSS) Annual Report 2009. National Perinatal Epidemiology Unit, Oxford 2009

Kumari AS.(2001) Pregnancy outcome in women with morbid obesity. *Int J GynecolObstet* **73**:101–7.

Langer O, Conway DL, Berkus MD et al (2000) A comparison of glyburide and insulin in women with gestational diabetes mellitus. *N Engl J Med*. **343**(16):1134-8

Larsen TB, Sorensen HT, Gislum M et al (2007) Maternal smoking, obesity and risk of venous thromboembolism during pregnancy and the puerperium: a population-based nested case-control study. *Thromb Res* **120**:505–9

Lewis, G (ed) 2007. *The Confidential Enquiry into Maternal and Child Health (CEMACH. Saving Mothers' Lives: reviewing maternal deaths to make motherhood safer – 2003-2005*. The Seventh Report on Confidential Enquiries into Maternal Deaths in the United Kingdom. **London**: CEMACH.

Lu GC, Rouse DJ, DuBard M, et al (2001) The effect of the increasing prevalence of maternal obesity on perinatal morbidity. *Am J Obstet Gynecol* **185**:845–9.

Magnussen EB, Vatten LJ, Lund-Nilsen TI, et al. (2007) Pre-pregnancy cardiovascular risk factors as predictors of PE: population based cohort study. *BMJ* **335**:978–81.

Maternal deaths in Australia 2000–2002. Australian Institute of Health and Welfare.

Available at: http://www.aihw.gov.au/publications/index.cfm/title/10207.

McColl MD, Ramsey JE, Tait RC et al. (1997) Risk factors for pregnancy associated venous thromboembolism. *Thromb Haemost* **78**:1183–8.

National Audit Office (2001) *Tackling Obesity in England.* Report by the Comptroller and Auditor General. London: Stationary Office.

National Collaborating Centre for Women's and Children's Health.(2008) Diabetes in pregnancy - management of diabetes and its complications from preconception to the postnatal period. Commissioned by National Institute for Health and Clinical Excellence. March 2008.

National Diabetes Data Group (1979) Classification and diagnosis of diabetes mellitus and other categories of glucose intolerance. *Diabetes* **28**: 1039–1057 *Nutrition* **13**; 807

National High Blood Pressure Education Program Working Group (1990) report on high blood pressure in pregnancy. *Am J Obstet Gynecol* **163**:1691–1712.

O'Brien TE, Ray JG, Chan W-S. (2003) Maternal Body mass index and risk of preeclampsia: a systematic review. *Epidemiology* **14**:368–74.

Poston L, Briley AL, Seed PT et al (2006). Vitamin C and vitamin E in pregnant women at risk for pre-eclampsia (VIP trial): randomised placebo-controlled trial . The Lancet 367:1145-1154

Rajasingam D, Seed PT, Briley AL et al (2009). A prospective study of pregnancy outcome and biomarkers of oxidative stress in nulliparous obese women. *Am J Obstet Gynecol.* **200**(4):395.e1-9

Roberts JM (1998) Endothelial dysfunction in PE. Semin Repro Endocrinol;**16**:5–15.

Rowan JA, Hague WM, Gao W et al (2008) for the MiG Trial Investigators. Metformin versus Insulin for the Treatment of Gestational Diabetes. *N Eng J Med* **358**:2003-15

Royal College of Obstetricians and Gynaecologists. (2004) Thromboprophylaxis During Pregnancy, Labour and After Vaginal Delivery. Green Top Guidelines. London: *RCOG.*

Royal College of Obstetricians and Gynaecologists. (2007) T*hromboembolic Disease in Pregnancy and the Puerperium: Acute Management.* Green Top Guidelines. London: *RCOG.*

Saving Mothers 2005-2007: Fourth Report on Confidential Enquiries into Maternal Deaths in South Africa. Government Printer, Petoria. Available at: http://www.doh.gov.za/docs/index.html (March 2010)

Sattar N, Clark P, Holmes A, et al (2001) Antenatal waist circumference and hypertension risk. *Obstet Gynecol* **97**:268–71.

Sattar N, Gaw A, Packard CJ, Greer IA. (1996) Potential pathogenic roles of aberrant lipoprotein and fatty acid metabolism in PE. *BJOG* **103**:614–20.

The HAPO Study Cooperative Research Group (2008) Hyperglycemia and adverse pregnancy outcomes. *N Eng J Med* **358**:1991-2002

Tsai AW, Cushman M, Rosamond WD, et al (2002) Cardiovascular risk factors and venous thromboembolism incidence: the longitudinal investigation of thromboembolism aetiology. *Arch Int Med* **162**:1182–9.

Vaya A, Falco C, Simo M, et al.(2007) Influence of lipids and obesity on haemorheological parameters in patients with deep vein thrombosis. *Thromb Haemost* **98**:621–6.

Watson K. (2007) Demographics, clinical outcome and audit of preconception care of women attending Guys and St Thomas' Foundation Trust diabetes antenatal service in 2007 Weiss JL, Malone FD, Emig D, et al (2004) Obesity, obstetric complications and caesarean delivery rate – a population-based screening study. *Am J Obstet Gynecol* **190**:1091–7.

Wolf M, Kettyle E, Sandler L, et al (2001) Obesity and PE: the potential role of inflammation. *Obstet Gynecol* **98**:757–62.

Chapter 7

Intrapartum Care of Obese women

Daghni Rajasingam and Sheela Swamy

Introduction

The growing obesity epidemic has resulted in increasing numbers of obese women requiring obstetric care and presenting unique challenges for their medical care providers (ACOG Committee Opinion 2005, Kumari 2001, Wolfe et al 1985, Robinson et al 2005). Antepartum and Intrapartum care represent a continuum. This chapter presents the challenges encountered during labour and delivery and the various dilemmas surrounding place and mode of delivery, intrapartum monitoring, analgesia and management of maternal and fetal complications.

Obesity related risk factors

Respiratory problems

There is a decreases in total lung capacity, vital capacity, inspiratory capacity and expiratory reserve volume in a morbidly obese pregnant woman thus leading to hypoxemia (Reisner et al 1999). These women should be evaluated for sleep aponea, and an assessment of pulmonary function should be undertaken where indicated. Oxygen saturations should be measured at the onset of labour as a baseline. Oxygen requirement increases in labour, particularly during the second stage, and can lead to decrease in maternal saturations and clinical symptoms of hypoxaemia. As labour leads to decrease in fetal oxygenation, maternal hypoxaemia in morbidly obese women further compromises fetal oxygenation. Hence fetal hypoxia may manifest more commonly prior to maternal hypoxia (Ramsey 1979).

Cardiovascular problems

In obese women cardiac output is considerably increased to help maintain adequate oxygenation. This leads to an increase in relative frequency of coronary artery disease compared to women with normal BMI. Maternal electrocardiogram and echocardiogram may be necessary when maternal cardiac status is being assessed antenatally in the morbidly obese women (Penderson 1992). Obesity is associated with increased stomach volume and increased acidity of gastric contents. These can lead to heart burn throughout pregnancy and aspiration of gastric contents can occur intrapartum if obese women receive a general anaesthetic. Horizontal positioning of the patient should be avoided.

Fetal growth

Obesity is associated with fetal macrosomia, leading to potential adverse maternal outcomes such as induction of labour, caesarean section, as well as adverse neonatal outcomes such as shoulder dystocia, birth injuries (Catelano 2007, Sheiner et al 2004, Yu et al 2006). Weiss et al (2004) aimed to determine whether obesity was associated with obstetric complications and caesarean deliveries. They studied a large, prospective, multicentre database from which 6102 patients were divided into three groups:
1. BMI 30 (control) comprising 3752 patients
2. BMI 30-34.9 (obese) comprising 1473 patients
3. BMI 35 or greater (morbidly obese) comprising 877 patients

Obesity and morbid obesity had a statistically significant association with fetal birth weight greater than 4000g (OR 1.7 and 1.9, respectively) and greater than 4500g (OR 2.0 and 2.4, respectively). Obesity and diabetes mellitus are independently associated with increased risk of macrosomic and large infants (Hoesberg at al 1993).

In obese women with hypertension there may be an increase in intrauterine growth retardation and regular growth scans are important. Fetal well-being should be monitored by repeated ultrasound scanning. Nutritional status of obese women, especially those from deprived areas, is also thought to contribute to poor fetal growth. In a study of obese women living in urban settings, Rajasingam et al (2009) found that there was a high incidence of fetal growth restriction in obese nulliparous women, but interestingly more than 50% was unrelated to developing pre eclampsia (PE).

Fetal distress and perinatal mortality

There is controversy in the literature regarding these outcomes. Indeed, maternal obesity has been linked to fetal distress, meconium aspiration, and perinatal mortality (Catelano 2007, Kristensen et al 2005). Kristensen et al (2005) evaluated the association between maternal prepregnancy BMI and the risk of still birth and neonatal death. Maternal obesity was associated with a more than doubled risk of still birth (OR 2.8, 95% CI 1.5-5.3) and neonatal death (OR 2.6, 95% CI1.2-5.8) compared with women with normal weight. No single cause of death explained the higher risk of perinatal mortality. In contrast Rhode et al (2005) found no differences between obese and nonobese women with regard to neonatal morbidity estimated by Apgar score, umbilical cord Ph, or admission to a neonatal intensive care unit.

In a large retrospective cohort study including 62 167 women within the Danish National Birth Cohort, the crude risks of PPROM (preterm premature rupture of membranes) and of induced preterm deliveries were higher in obese women than in normal weight women, especially before 34 completed weeks of gestation. In the preterm prediction study by Brost et al (1997), the authors were able to show a linear relationship between increasing prepregnancy BMI and increasing caesarean delivery.

Birthing considerations for obese women.

Equipment

There is no consensus regarding the safest mode of delivery for the obese mother and the fetus. Any unit caring for obese and severely obese patients should have equipment designed for obese patients in order to provide adequate care. These include appropriate size dressing gowns, extra large BP monitors, wide chairs and automated beds to support the weight and width of obese patients. Medical and surgical teams must be aware of the potential need for High Dependancy Unit (HDU) and or intensive care unit (ICU) (Whittemore et al 2005).

Mode and place of birth

When the balance of risk favours a vaginal delivery, clinicians should attempt to avoid unnecessary interventions such as induction of labour. The obese patient should be encouraged to attend antenatal classes and in cases where this may not be possible every effort should be made to provide community based support to increase her awareness regarding labour process, analgesia, positions for labour and delivery. Upon arrival in the labour unit, presentation of the fetus should be confirmed by ultrasound scan, if possible, as obesity is associated with malpresentation. One-to-one midwifery support should be provided during labour. Venous access should be secured early and in cases of difficulty, peripheral venous access should be attempted by anaesthetic personnel.

Induction of labour

Induction rates are generally higher in overweight women (Sebire 2001, Bhattacharya et al 2007). Induction of labour is not a benign process, it increases intervention rate in itself. A study (Kariu and Raynor 2004) of 5 131 women showed an increase in the incidence of failed induction in both overweight women (P<0.001) and women who had gained more than one unit of BMI during pregnancy (P < 0.001). Obesity per se is not an indication for induction of labour.

Monitoring in labour

The guidelines for electronic fetal monitoring are equally applicable for a slim or obese patients. However, external monitoring may be difficult and more challenging for the midwifery personnel attending to the obese patient. This may lead to artificial rupture of membranes being undertaken, in the absence of a real indication, and a fetal scalp electrode being placed. Anxiety about fetal monitoring increases intervention. Apart from the loss of mechanical protection (Mergoni 1988), it results in introduction of infectious micro organisms, with consequences that have been described in retrospect (Iffy et al 1979, Apuzzio et al 1982, Scott et al 1994) but remain far too often unconsidered.

The advantage of fetal scalp electrode monitoring in the obese patient outweighs the potential risks. Sometimes intermittent auscultation is an alternative option. Ultrasound location of fetal heart prior to intermittent auscultation may be of benefit. The presence of a scalp electrode on an already delivered fetal scalp may reassure the midwife and clinician to await restitution and further contraction prior to attempting delivery of shoulders (Stenchever, Gittens-Williams 2006, Ramiere et al 2006, Stallings et al 2001).

Intrapartum variables of labour monitoring as well as anaesthetic and neonatal variables were compared between 50 morbidly obese and 50 normal weight women. The morbidly obese group was observed to be significantly more prone to invasive fetal monitoring (27% vs. 0%), difficult uterine contraction monitoring (30% vs. 0%), and more medical personnel involvement (22% vs. 2%). They were also found to be more likely to experience multiple epidural attempts (28% vs. 0 %,), complications in labour (32% vs. 6%) and paediatric involvement (26% vs. 3%) (Catelano 2007).

Vaginal birth after caesarean section (VBAC)

Obesity reduces the chances of successful VBAC after one previous lower segment caesarean section. In a study of 1213 women whose first child had been delivered by lower-segment caesarean section, the success rate for VBAC was 77.2% overall (Juhasz 2005). The study reported success rates for women with (P <0.001):

- BMI <19 were 83.1%
- BMI <19-26 were 79.9%
- BMI<26-29 were 69.3%
- BMI > 29 were 68.2%

Women who gained more than 18kg during pregnancy had a VBAC success rate of 66.8%, while those who gained < 18kg had a success rate of 79.1%. (P <0.001).

In another study of 510 women attempting VBAC, a success rate of 54.6 % was achieved in obese women compared with 70.5% in women of normal BMI (P=0.003) (Durnwald et al 2004). A cohort of 69 women each with a prepregnancy weight of over 135kg had a VBAC success rate of just 13%, compared with a success rate of 57.1% in 70 women of 90-135kg and 81.8% in 70 women weighing less than 90 kg prepregnancy (Carroll et al 2003).

Anaesthesia

Obesity is a risk factor for anaesthesia related maternal mortality. Morbidly obese women must be considered as high risk and deserve an anaesthetic consultation during their antenatal care. The significant difficulty in administering epidural analgesia should not preclude their use in labour. A more liberalised use of regional techniques may be a means to further reduce anaesthesia-related maternal mortality in the obese population. The mother's life should not be jeopardised to save a compromised fetus. Prophylactic placement of an epidural catheter when not contraindicated in labouring morbidly obese women would potentially decrease anaesthetic and perinatal complications associated with attempts at emergency provision of regional or general anaesthesia. Early mobilisation, aggressive chest physiotherapy and adequate pain control are essential components of effective postoperative care (Saravanakumar et al 2006). Obese women are not only at high risk of airway complications, cardiopulmonary dysfunction, perioperative morbidity and mortality but also pose technical challenges. Obesity also influences the fetal outcomes. Increasing use of regional techniques contributes to the reduced anaesthesia-related maternal mortality. Preconception counselling, antenatal screening and anaesthetic assessment are strongly encouraged. They were also found to be more likely to experience multiple epidural attempts (28% vs. 0%, p<0.001), complications in labour (32% vs. 6%, p < 0.001) and paediatric involvement (26% vs. 3%, OR for 95% confidence interval is 1.5-20.8) (Rayet al 2008).

Intrapartum complications in obese women

Obesity increases the rates of all types of complications during delivery. During labour there is a delay in the emptying of the stomach where food and fluids may remain there for several hours. Consuming food while in labour was generally discouraged in the past but light easily digestable foods and non-aerated drinks are probably more help than harm. A prospective randomised controlled trial conducted in a birth centre in a London teaching hospital investigated the effect of feeding during labour on obstetric and neonatal outcomes. It concluded that consumption of a light diet during labour did not influence obstetric or neonatal outcomes in participants, nor did it increase the incidence of vomiting. Women who are allowed to eat in labour have similar lengths of labour and operative delivery rates to those allowed water only (Geraldine O' Sulivan et al 2009). Women should be given ranitidine tablets 150 mgs at eight hourly intervals in labour.

In the event of needing a general anaesthetic, there is a risk of aspiration and the acid contents of the stomach may cause bronchiolar spasm and pneumonia (Mendelson's syndrome). Women should receive IV Ranitidine 50 mg, IV Metoclopramide 10 mg, and 30mls of oral Sodium Citrate prior to a general anaesthetic. They should also be encouraged to adopt the position that leads to the least respiratory compromise. Routine positions like lithotomy, Trendelenberg, and McRoberts positions may not be easily tolerated by obese women. In addition respiratory compromise may also obscure the signs of shock, pulmonary embolism and amniotic fluid embolism.

Positional abnormalities such a malrotation, asynclitism of head, deflexion are the same for a morbidly obese women as for a normal weight patient. However in the presence of fetal macrosomia, primary and secondary arrest in first stage of labour is quite common. In such cases perseverance of trial of labour is not justifiable due to the increased incidence of shoulder dystocia and perinatal morbidity.

There is controversy about abdominal breech delivery in obese women. As operative delivery involves risks in obese women, a small minority of experts believe in allowing multiparous women with an estimated fetal weight on ultrasound scan to try for a vaginal breech delivery. However due to risks involved with obstetric anaesthesia, and the rapid need for delivery in the event of fetal distress, an elective abdominal breech delivery is recommended to obese primiparous women by majority of obstetricians.

Management of first stage of labour

One-to-one midwifery care should be the gold standard in labour. The woman and her partner should be kept well informed of the current stage of labour and cervical dilatation. Women should be encouraged to remain mobile and well hydrated during early stages of labour. Special birthing balls or a special birthing stool may prove to be a useful aid to the birthing process. This keeps the obese patient in upright position, leading to less respiratory compromise, and gravity may aid labour progress. Women should be encouraged to pass urine every two hours in labour, and if urinary retention is suspected, an in-and-out catheter should be used. A Modified Early Warning Trigger Chart should be maintained and regular observations recorded.

Management of second stage of labour

Operative delivery

The increase in caesarean deliveries in obese women is of great concern because of the potential operative and post operative morbidity, especially when compared with that associated with vaginal delivery. Crane et al (1997) studied a population of 20 130 women with live births stratified by maternal prepregnancy BMI to compare route of delivery. The study found the rate of caesarian delivery was:
- 20.2% in women with BMI>29 (designated as non-obese)
- 30.1% in women with a BMI between 29 and 34.9
- 38.6% in women with a BMI between 35 and 39.9
- 45.9% in women with BMI exceeding 39.9

Current rates of CS vary from 29% in the USA (Cunningham et al 2005) and even higher in the South American continent. Kaiser and Kirby (2001) demonstrated an odds ratio of 3.99 for the risk of caesarean delivery in a low risk obese population of women managed by midwives. These low risk healthy obese women were defined as those without chronic conditions (diabetes, hypertension and unstable asthma), prenatal conditions (multiple gestations, fetal malformations and gestational diabetes), and those who chose a repeat caesarean delivery.

Vaginal examination should be performed to confirm full dilatation of the cervix. In the absence of strong urges to push it is safe to allow 1-2 hours for the descent of fetal head prior to commencing active pushing. The length of second stage of labour should be discussed with the mother so she is aware of the rational for passive second stage. National UK (NICE 2007) guidance on the management of second stage of labour maximum suggests maximum duration of second stage is as follows:

	Epidural	No epidural
Primip	4 hours	3 hours
Multip	3 hours	2 hours

Obese women tend to have a sedentary lifestyle compared to normal weight women and increase in weight during pregnancy further restricts their mobility which has implications in both the first and second stage of labour. The woman should adopt a position most suited to her in order to push effectively, along with some assistance from gravity. Avoid supine position as this worsens respiratory problems in the mother and causes hypotension which in turn leads to fetal heart rate abnormalities. A sitting, squatting or 'all fours' position is quite often acceptable, causing the least respiratory compromise to the obese mother.

Delivery of the head

In the presence of, or in anticipation of shoulder dystocia, a generous episiotomy may be useful to gain access to perform internal measures to deliver the anterior shoulder.

Fetal head on most occasions rotates to occipitotransverse position during the course of the same contraction. If there is a loop of cord around the fetal neck , attempt to slip it over the head if loose. Traditionally it was recommended the cord be clamped with two pairs of artery forceps and divided between them if tight around the fetal neck. This procedure should not be practiced routinely as this may lead to catastrophic consequences in the presence of shoulder dystocia if vaginal delivery fails (Stenchever,

Gittens- Williams 2006, Ramieri et al 2006). Minimal easing of an unduly tight cord permits continued circulation between the placenta and the fetus. Darkening of the fetal head is a normal phenomenon due to impaired skin circulation which will be re-established soon after delivery of the shoulders and body.

On occasions, the fetal head remains in occipitoanterior position and the head retracts towards the perineum, a phenomenon known as 'turtle sign'. This is a sign of shoulder dystocia. Lack of restitution should prepare the attendants for potential shoulder dystocia.

Delivery of shoulders

If 'turtle sign' is seen, or shoulders have not delivered after delivery of fetal head despite gentle traction, the midwife or obstetrician should immediately consider shoulder dystocia as a possible cause. They should immediately call for help and institute emergency procedures for shoulder dystocia.

The incidence of shoulder dystocia is generally reported to be between 0.5 % and 1.5% in the general pregnant population. Fetal macrosomia is the most significant risk factor for shoulder dystocia and hence obese women are prime candidates.

Incidence varies by birth weight:
- 0.3-1% in infants weighing 2500 – 4000 grams
- 5-7% in infants weighing 4000 – 4500 grams
- 8-10% in infants weighing > 4500 grams
- > 50% occur in normal weight infants.

Acker (1985) found that babies weighing over 4500gms experienced shoulder dystocia 22.6% of the time.

Next to macrosomia, the factor most closely associated with shoulder dystocia is maternal diabetes in pregnancy. Babies of diabetic mothers had a three-to-four fold increase in the risk of shoulder dystocia compared to babies of non diabetic mothers in each weight category (Acker 1985). Although diabetic mothers accounted for only 1.4% of the birth population in this study, they accounted for 4.9% of shoulder dystocias. Acker also showed that although the general rate of Erb's palsy following shoulder dystocia is roughly 10%, 17% of babies born to diabetic mothers developed Erb's palsy.

Fetal hypoxia is a potential serious complication of shoulder dystocia. It can lead to permanent neurological damage or even death. Once the head is delivered the umbilical cord is compressed between the fetal body and the maternal pelvis. Fetal pH is said to drop at a rate of 0.04 per minute. In a noncompromised fetus, it takes seven minutes for the pH to drop from 7.25

to 6.97. Resuscitation of these neonates becomes increasingly difficult as persistent fetal circulation becomes more common.

Surgery

For surgery on obese patients, additional personnel needed for delivery include a senior obstetrician and anaesthetist. Delivery should be timed if elective operative delivery is considered when additional clinicians are available for assistance. Additional support staff to aid in obstetric emergencies and assist surgical procedures should be organised.

During labour, the patient must be positioned to promote easy ventilation without compromising surgical access. Left lateral positioning should be used in all patients to improve venous return to heart. Pneumatic Compression Devices (PCD) should be used as prophylaxis.

Abdominal incisions

The appropriate placement of abdominal incisions is of particular concern in obese patients. One must weigh the benefits of improved access against the complications associated with wound closure and wound disruption. Transverse incisions are often favoured as they provide best cosmetic result and the strength is superior to that of a vertical incision. Pfannensteil and Maylard's incisions (Burke, Gallup 2003) are commonly used incisions in obstetric surgery. Both these incisions have the disadvantage of providing an awkward exposure particularly in obese patients. These incisions are usually placed in the skin folds of the panniculus, where it might increase infectious morbidity (Houston, Raynor 2000). Vertical incisions provide the best exposure, allow rapid entry, less haemorrhage and haematoma rate (Burke, Gallup 2003, Houston, Raynor 2000, Grantcharov, Rosenberg 2001). Wall et al (2003) conducted a retrospective cohort study of 239 women with a BMI greater than 35 undergoing primary caesarean delivery. The overall incidence of wound complications was 12% which is comparable to that in other studies. The incidence of wound complications in patients with vertical compared with transverse incisions was significantly higher (35% vs. 9%). Decision for site of abdominal incision should be made appropriate to individual's body habitus, urgency of the procedure and prior abdominal incisions.

Abdominal closure

A suture with delayed absorption should be used for the fascial closure.

Midline surgical incisions should be closed with a mass closure technique. Subcutaneous tissue layer should be closed with interrupted sutures if the layer exceeds 3 cms.

Consider use of staples or interrupted sutures for skin closure. Pelvic and subrectus drains should be considered to allow drainage of blood and these should be removed after 24 to 48 hours when patient is mobilising. These may also help to detect any ongoing intra-abdominal haemorrhage as clinical signs may not be obvious in obese patients.

Infections

Infectious complications are the leading cause of operative and post operative morbidity in patients undergoing caesarean delivery (Houston, Raynor 2000). Infectious morbidity includes wound infections and endometritis, both leading to increased hospital stay and patient dissatisfaction. In obese patients, caesarean delivery is associated with an eight fold increase in infectious morbidity compared with vaginal delivery (Lang, King 2008).

Prophylactic antibiotics should be given for all caesarean deliveries as it reduces the infectious morbidity by 75%. Standard doses are adequate in achieving adequate tissue levels in majority of patients, however in morbidly obese patients, dosing should be individualised. Manual removal of placenta and repair of third and fourth degree tears should in addition receive broad spectrum antibiotics for additional five days. Additional antibiotics should be considered in the event of a blood loss of greater than 1500 ml or if the operative time exceeds three hours (Forse et al 1989).

Post operative care

Post operative recovery should be optimised by providing HDU care with adequate monitoring of respiratory and cardiac function. ITU care may be necessary in case of respiratory compromise and haemodynamic instability. Most patients can be managed in standard maternity units with early mobilisation and support from physiotherapists.

The Royal College of Obstetricians and Gynaecologists ([RCOG] 2009) guidelines on thromboprophylaxis during pregnancy and labour, and after normal vaginal delivery, recommend that as obesity (BMI over 30 or weight 90 kg) is an important independent risk factor for post partum venous thromboembolism (VTE), even after vaginal delivery, the combination of obesity with any other risk factor for VTE should lead to thromboprophylaxis with low molecular weight heparin (LMWH) for 3-5 days postpartum or until discharge in women who are hospitalised for a longer period of time. Thromboprophylaxis should be considered for up to six weeks in the morbidly obese women.

Early mobilisation with guidance from physiotherapist is recommended. Patients should be encouraged to use support devices available to mobilise in and out of bed and bath to encourage independence.

Obese women should receive counselling regarding importance of hygiene and wound care. Daily inspection of perineum or abdominal wounds should be undertaken by the care providers. Close follow up after discharge should be ensured to detect infection and institute appropriate treatment. Early referral to the unit should be made if infection is suspected for patient assessment and treatment to prevent systemic infection. A post caesarean wound infection may take one of two forms, wound cellulitis or abscess: The Vacuum Assisted Closure (VAC) system can be used for patients with postoperative abdominal wound dehiscences that could not be closed immediately and who were at high risk for healing complications.

Conclusion

Obesity is an increasing problem in economically advanced countries and in the developing world. It is a risk factor for many untoward intrapartum and postpartum events, hence poses a challenge to maternity teams. Vigilance, anticipation, preparation and appropriate management are required to ensure safe delivery of obese patient and the fetus. Clinicians should remember that the postpartum period is the ideal time to discuss future contraception and weight loss so weight retention in one pregnancy is not carried onto the next. The postnatal period of one pregnancy could be the preconceptual period of the subsequent pregnancy. Obese women should be aware of their risks and be involved in decisions regarding their care.

References

Acker DB, Sachs BP, Friedman EA. (1985) Risk factors for shoulder dystocia. *Obstet Gynecol.* **66**:762–8. 13.

ACOG Committee Opinion 314 (2005) Obesity in pregnancy. *Obstet Gynecol* **106**: 671-5.

Apuzzio J, Iffy L (1985) *Perinatal infection control.* In: Keith LG, ed. Infections in Reproductive Health. Vol 1, Common Infections. Lancaster, UK: MTP Press, 171-84.

Apuzzio JJ, Reyelt C, Pelosi M et al (1982). Prophylactic antibiotics for caesarean section: comparison of high-and low-risk patients for endomyometritis. *Obstet Gynecol* **59**:693-8.

Brost BC, Goldenberg RL, Mercer BM, et al.(1997) The preterm prediction study: association of caesarean delivery with increases in maternal weight and body mass index. *Am J Obstet Gynaecol* **177**:333-41.

Bhattacharya S, Campbell DM, Liston WA, et al (2007) Effect of body mass index on pregnancy outcomes in nulliparous women delivering singleton babies. *BMC Public health* **7:**168.

Burke JJ, Gallup DG. (2003) *Incisions for gynaecologic surgery.* In: Operative Gynecology, 9th edn Philadelphia: Lippincott Williams and Wilkins:256-90.

Carroll CS, Magann EF, Chauhan SP, et al.(2003)Vaginal birth after caesarean section versus elective repeat caesarean delivery: weight-based outcomes. *Am J Obstet Gynecol* **188**:1516-20.

Catelano PM (2007) Management of obesity in pregnancy. *Obstet Gynaecol* **109**:419-33

Durnwald CP, Ethrenberg HM, Mercer BM. *(*2004) The impact of maternal obesity and weight gain on vaginal birth after caesarean section success. *Am J Obstet Gynecol* **191**:954-7.

Forse RA, Karam B, Mclean LD, et al (1989)Antibiotic prophylaxis for surgery in morbidly obese patients. *Surgery;* **106**:750-6.

Garite TJ, Spellacy WN. (1994) *Premature rupture of membranes.* In: Scott JR, DiSaia PJ, Hammond CB, Spellacy WN, eds. Danforth's Obestetrics and Gynecology, 7th edn. Philadelphia: JB Lippincott, :305-16.

O'Sullivan G, Liu B, Hart D (2009) Effect of food intake during labour on obstetric outcome: randomised controlled trial. March 24: 10.1136/bmj.b784.

Grantcharov TP, Rosenberg J. (2001)Vertical compared with transverse incisions in abdominal surgery. *Eur J Surg* **167**:260-7.

Hoesberg B, Gruppuso PA, Coustan DR.(1993) Hyperinsulinaemia in macrosomic infants of nondiabetic mothers. *Diabetes Care*; **16**:32-6.

Houston MC, Raynor BD. (2000) Postoperative morbidity in the morbidly obese patient: supraumbilical and low transverse abdominal approaches. *Am J Obstet Gynecol*; **182**:1033-5.

Iffy L, Kaminetzky HA, Maidman JE, at al. (1979) Control of perinatal infections with traditional preventive measures. *Obstet Gynecol* **54**:403-11.

Iffy L, Apuzzio JJ, Mitra S, et al (1994). Rates of caesarean section and perinatal outcome: perinatal mortality. *Acta Obstet Gynaecol Scand* **73**:225-30.81

Juhasz G, Gyamfi C, Gyamfi P, et al. (2005) Effect of body mass index and excessive weight gain on success of vaginal birth after caesarean delivery. *Obstet Gynecol* **106**:741-6.

Kabiru W, Raynor BD.(2004) Obstetric outcomes associated with increase in BMI category during pregnancy. *Am J Obstet Gynecol* **191**:928-32.

Kaiser PS, Kirby RS. (2001)Obesity as a risk factor for caesarean in low – risk population.

Obstet Gynecol **97**:39-43.

Kleigman RM, Gross T. (1985) Perinatal problems of the obese mother and her infant. *Obstet Gynecol* **66**:299-305.

Kristensen J, Vestergaard M, Wisborg K, et al. (2005) Pre-pregnancy weight and the risk of still birth and neonatal death. *Br J Obstet Gynaecol*; **112**:403-8.

Kumari AS. (2001)Pregnancy outcome in women with morbid obesity. *Int J Obstet Gynaecol* **73**:101-7.

Lang CT, King JC. (2008) Maternal mortality in the united states. *Best pract Res Clin Obstet Gynaecol 2008* (Epub ahead of print)

Penderson H, Santos AC, Finster M. (1992)A*naesthesia in the high-risk patient.* In: Reece EA, Hobbins JC, Mahoney MJ, Petrie RH, eds. Medicine of the Fetus and the Mother. Philadelphia: JB Lippincott, :1482-93.

Mergoni A. La Legge di Pascal e il torchio pelvico nel meccanismo fisiologico del parto. Minerva Ginecol 1988; 40:199-214.

National Institute for Clinical Effectiveness Guidance, Intrapartum care: Care of Healthy women and their babies during childbirth, 26 September 2007. Available at www.nice.org.uk

Rajasingam D, Seed PT, Briley AL et al (2009) A prospective study of pregnancy outcome and biomarkers of oxidative stress in nulliparous obese women. *Am J Obstet Gynecol.* **200**(4):395.e1-9

Ramieri K, Iffy L. (2006) *Shoulder dystocia.* In: Appuzio JJ, Vintzileos MA, Iffy L, eds. Operative Obstetrics 3rd edn. London: Taylor & Francis :253-63.

Ramsey EM. (1979) Anatomy and pathology of uteroplacental circulation. In:Kaminetzky HA, Iffy L, eds. New Techniques and concepts in Maternal and Fetal Medicine. New York: Van Nostrand Reinhold :7-19.

Ray A, Hildreth A, Esen UI (2008) Morbid Obesity and Intrapartum care. *J Obstet Gynaecol.* **28**(3):301-4.

Reisner LS, Nichols KP. (1999)*Anaesthetic considerations for complicated pregnancies.* In:Creasy RK, Resnik R, EDS. Maternal-Fetal Medicine, 4th edn. Philadelphia: WB Saunders:1215-32

Robinson HE, O'Connell CM, Joseph KS, et al. (2005) Maternal outcomes in pregnancies complicated by obesity. *Obstet Gynecol* **106**:1357-64.

Rode L, Nilas L, Wojedmann K, (2005)Tabo neonatal death. *Br J Obstet Gynaecol* **112**:403-8.r

Rode L, Nilas L, Wojedmann K, Tabo neonatal death. Br J Obstet Gynaecol2005; 112:403-8.r.A.

Royal College of Obstetricians and Gynaecologists (RCOG) (2009) RCOG Green Top Guidelines, No. 37, Nov 2009

Saravanakumar K, Rao SG, Cooper GM; Anaesthesia. 2006,Jan; 61(1):36-48. (1):36-48.

Sebire NJ, Jolly M, Harris JP, et al. (2005) Maternal obesity and pregnancy outcome: a study of

287,213 pregnancies in London. *Int J Obes Relat Metab Disord* **25**:1175-82

Sheiner E, Levy A, Menes TS, et al. (2004) Maternal obesity as an independent risk factor for caesarean delivery. *Paediatr Perinat Epidemiol* **18**:196-201.

Stallings SP, Edwards RK, Johnson JWC. (2001) Correlation of head-to-body delivery intervals in shoulder dystocia and umbilical artery acidosis. *Am J Obstet Gynecol* **185**:268-7.

Stenchever SF, Gittens-Williams LN. (2006) *Normal vaginal delivery*. In: Apuzzio JJ, Vintzileos MA, Iffy L, eds. Operative Obstetrics, 3rd edn. London: Taylor & Francis 241-52.

Royal College Of Obstetricians and Gynaecologists. *Thromboprophylaxis during Pregnancy, Labour and after vaginal delivery*. RCOG Guideline No. 37. London: Available at: www.rcog.org.uk

Wall PD, Deucy EE, Glantz JC, et al. (2003)Vertical skin incisions and wound complications in the obese patient. *Obstet Gynecol* **102**;952-6.

Weiss JL, Malone FD, Emig D, et al. (2004)FASTER research consortium. Obesity, obstetric complications and caesarean delivery rate: a population based screening study. *Am j Obstet Gynaecol* **190**:1091-7.

Whittemore AD, Kelly J, Shikora s, et al.(2005) Specialised staff and equipment for weight loss surgery patients: best practice guidelines. *Obes Res* **13**:283-9.

Wolfe HM, Gross TL, Sokol RJ, et al. (1988) Determinants of morbidity in obese women delivered by caesarean. *Obstetr Gynecol* **71**:691-6.

Yu CK, Teoh TG, Robinson S. (2006) Obesity in pregnancy. *Br J Obstet Gynaecol* **113**:1117-25

Chapter 8

Anaesthetic Management of the Obese Parturient

Rory Bell and Jason Cronje

Introduction

The Confidential Enquiry into Maternal and Child Health (CEMACH) has shown a welcome reduction in anaesthetic related deaths over the years despite a considerable increase in the number of women delivered by caesarean section (CS). Anaesthesia for CS is now 36 times safer than it was in the 1960's and six times safer than in the 1982–1984 triennium (Cooper 2005). Despite this, anaesthesia still poses a risk to pregnant women.

The CEMACH 2003–2005 reported six deaths directly related to anaesthesia and of these four were obese (CEMACH 2007). A remarkably similar association was reported from North America where eight of a series of 855 maternal deaths were related to anaesthesia and six of these were obese (Mhyre 2007). It is also worth noting that regardless of which side of the Atlantic these tragedies unfolded on, the majority of these deaths occurred postoperatively following general anaesthesia (GA).

There are several reasons for this excess morbidity and mortality in obese parturients. Both pregnancy and obesity cause significant changes in the mother's anatomy, physiology and pharmacology. There are also substantial practical difficulties associated with the anaesthetic management of the obese parturient. Finally these women are more likely to require anaesthetic intervention because of the obstetric difficulties presented by obesity (Cedergren 2004). At least two out of every three morbidly obese women on the delivery suite will require the services of an anaesthetist (McCrae 2009).

Anatomy and physiology

Respiratory system

The maintenance of a clear airway is the cornerstone of safe anaesthetic practice. Uncorrected loss of the airway will inevitably result in death secondary to hypoxia. Tracheal intubation is required for CS under general anaesthesia not only to facilitate ventilation, but also to protect the airway from the aspiration of gastric contents. Asphyxia secondary to loss of the airway or pneumonitis following aspiration of gastric acid were the main reasons for anaesthetic mortality for many years. Such catastrophes are now thankfully rare due to improvements in anaesthetic practice such as a reduction in the GA rate, restricted oral intake in labour, antacid prophylaxis, intubation aids, better training and monitoring.

The incidence of failed endotracheal intubation remains, however, increased from 1:2-3000 in the general population compared to 1:250 in the obstetric population (Hawthorne et al 1996). Similarly the incidence of difficult intubation is increased from 2.2% in lean patients (BMI <30) to 15.5% in the obese (Juvin et al 2003) and may be up to 33% in the morbidly obese parturient (Hood and Dewan 1993). The combination of pregnancy and obesity may therefore create serious problems with intubation which may in turn lead to hypoxia of both mother and fetus. Difficult or failed intubation will also put the mother at risk of aspiration of gastric contents.

Both pregnancy and obesity decrease the body's oxygen stores when lying flat and increase the rate at which those stores are consumed. It is therefore unsurprising that oxygen desaturation occurs three times more quickly in the obese than the non obese pregnant patient (McClelland et al 2009). Inducing anaesthesia in the semi recumbent 'ramped' position has been shown to improve intubating conditions and delay the onset of hypoxia in obese patients (Collins et al 2004).

Airway and breathing problems do not end with a successful intubation. Obesity is associated with difficulties in ventilation related to a reduction in chest wall compliance, displacement of the endotracheal tube and bronchospasm. As mentioned above the largest subgroup of maternal anaesthetic deaths in recent studies has involved the postoperative loss of the airway following GA in obese women (CEMACH 2007; Mhyre 2007).

Cardiovascular system

Obesity predisposes to cardiac co-morbidity as illustrated in *Table 8.1*. Any cardiac morbidity will be stressed by the increased work of the raised cardiac output seen in both obesity and pregnancy.

Acute physiological cardiovascular changes may occur with the exaggerated aortocaval compression from the obese abdomen. In morbidly obese parturients with a well developed panniculus ('apron') caution must be exercised when retracting the panniculus. Sudden aortocaval and chest compression can cause rapid severe maternal cardiac decompensation which may in turn cause maternal or fetal demise (Hodgkinson and Husain 1980; Tsueda et al 1979). The panniculus will often need to be moved to achieve surgical access for a CS but this must be done slowly and may require suspension to reduce the weight on the mother's chest.

Co-existing disease

Obesity is associated with a number of medical conditions, many of which increase the risks of anaesthesia and surgery. See *Table 8.1* below.

Pharmacology

Many anaesthetic drug doses are calculated according to bodyweight. It is often unclear if this is the correct approach in obesity. It may be more appropriate to calculate certain drugs doses bases on ideal or lean bodyweight.

Many sedative, anaesthetic and analgesic drugs are lipophilic; in other words they readily dissolve in fat. It will therefore take longer for these drugs to be metabolised and cleared from the body. Obese patients show sensitivity to opiate analgesic drugs especially if they have obstructive sleep apnoea. The resulting sedation and respiratory depression on a background

Table 8.1 Diseases associated with obesity	
Condition	**Interaction with anaesthesia**
Asthma	Bronchospasm especially during or after GA
Obstructive sleep apnoea	Associated with difficult ventilation and intubation. Pulmonary hypertension, arrhythmias, sudden death. Postoperative airway obstruction. Risks to baby.
Hypertension	Labile blood pressure. Pre eclampsia. Cardiac morbidity
Ischaemic heart disease	Important cause of maternal death
Cardiomyopathy	Important cause of maternal death
Thromboembolism	Deep vein thrombosis, Pulmonary embolism. Effects of anticoagulation
Wound infection	Sepsis, haemodynamic instability

of reduced reserve may precipitate respiratory failure in these patients.

Respiratory depression in these patients may cause oxygen desaturation, airway obstruction and impaired cough.

Intramuscular injections may actually be deposited in the less vascular subcutaneous fat which will lead to slower and unpredictable absorption of the drug.

Opioid labour analgesia is therefore not ideal in the obese parturient as it may be slow to act but will persist for much longer than in a non obese woman. Opioids also exacerbate the delayed gastric emptying of labour and therefore put these women at even greater risk of pulmonary aspiration of gastric contents should a general anaesthetic be required.

In contrast epidural and spinal anaesthesia may be more effective in the obese as the available volume of the epidural and spinal space is reduced by fat. Obese patients will, therefore, have a more extensive block for a given dose of local anaesthetic than the non obese. Regional analgesia will not reduce gastric emptying.

Practical problems

The practical anaesthetic management of obese women for both vaginal and operative delivery is often challenging.

Simple interventions such as intravenous (IV) cannulation can become a protracted struggle especially in the morbidly obese where veins may be both invisible and impalpable under the deep subcutaneous fat. Halfway through a major postpartum haemorrhage is not the time to be discovering this and it is therefore good practice to secure IV access early in any morbidly obese patient.

Measurement of blood pressure is important in these patients but may prove technically difficult or unreliable. An undersized cuff will overestimate the blood pressure. Extra large cuffs must be available to ensure reliable readings but even these may be difficult to position on large conical upper arms. Frequent measurement of blood pressure during anaesthesia may necessitate insertion of an arterial line for direct arterial pressure monitoring.

Insertion of a spinal or epidural can be similarly difficult and this is one reason why it is essential that the duty anaesthetist is informed of all morbidly obese women when they are admitted to the delivery suite. Difficulty palpating bony landmarks, false loss of resistance in fat pockets and the greater depth of the epidural space all conspire to challenge the anaesthetist. As a result, more than one attempt at epidural insertion may be required in as many as 75% of morbidly obese women with 14% requiring more than three attempts (Perlow and Morgan 1994). Even when apparently successfully sited, up to 42% of these epidurals may fail (Hood and Dewan 1993). Failure of epidural labour analgesia must be acted on promptly as attempting to "top up" an inadequate epidural for an emergency CS can cause a dangerous delay in delivery of the baby, excess spread of subsequent spinal anaesthesia, or emergency general anaesthesia.

A range of bariatric equipment is necessary for the safe care of obese patients. Many older operating tables with manual controls are rated to approximately 135 kg. If this weight is exceeded there is a danger that the table will not raise, lower or tilt. Such a failure could lead to, or compound, a major untoward incident. A further advantage of bariatric tables is the availability of extension pieces to widen the platform sufficiently to accommodate the increased physical size of bariatric women. All units should therefore have immediate access to an appropriately weight rated operating table and extension pieces.

At CS, retraction of the pannus is difficult but may often be achieved with long wide strips of elastoplast anchored to the side of the operating table. This can, as discussed above, lead to significant cardiovascular compromise. Some authors have therefore suggested retraction combined with elevation (Whitty et al 2006).

Management

Antenatal assessment

The CEMACH recommends that all morbidly obese pregnant women are assessed by an anaesthetist in the antenatal period. Anaesthetic assessment involves taking a medical, obstetric and anaesthetic history. Women should particularly be asked about significant co-morbidities such as asthma, hypertension, thromboembolism, diabetes and cardiac disease. Information regarding difficulties with previous anaesthetics and operations should be sought.

Examination of the cardiovascular and respiratory system including documentation of heart rate, blood pressure and oxygen saturation is helpful. The anaesthetist can also assess the risk of peripartum anaesthetic problems by looking at the mother's airway, back and veins.

Depending on clinical findings, investigations such as ECG, echocardiography, lung function or sleep studies may be indicated.

Management plan

A specific management plan will be tailored to the individual patient after discussion with the multidisciplinary team.

For reasons outlined above, the overriding anaesthetic concern is to avoid being caught unprepared for emergency general anaesthesia.

The duty anaesthetist must, therefore, be made aware of all morbidly obese women in the delivery suite or otherwise at risk of anaesthetic intervention. Senior anaesthetic input should be sought if there are any concerns.

The anaesthetic of choice for CS is a combined spinal epidural (CSE) which combines the reliability of a spinal block with the facility to "top up" via the epidural catheter if surgery is prolonged or complicated. The epidural needle also provides a useful guide for the spinal needle. Extra long spinal and/or epidural needles may occasionally be required. Ultrasound can facilitate successful epidural insertion in obese parturients with impalpable landmarks by enabling identification of the midline, spinous processes and depth of the epidural space (Arzola et al 2007).

Nil by mouth policies during labour are controversial and differ between units. Obese women are at increased risk of operative intervention, general anaesthesia, difficult intubation and aspiration of gastric contents. They must therefore be restricted to clear fluids only during labour. Similarly they should receive regular oral antacid prophylaxis.

An early epidural in labour ensures good analgesia, attenuates the physiological stress of labour and avoids the considerable side effects of intramuscular opioids. If properly monitored during labour it may also provide anaesthesia for any surgical interventions.

Postpartum care must include careful assessment for thromboprophylaxis with graduated elastic compression stockings and an appropriately increased dose of low molecular weight heparin. Good hydration and early mobilisation are important.

Obese women who undergo operative intervention need extended recovery facilities with appropriately trained staff. Good postoperative analgesia and chest physiotherapy is essential for those who have had general anaesthesia or have coexisting respiratory disease (Saravanakumar, 2006). Those with obstructive sleep apnoea, respiratory or cardiac disease will require HDU care.

References

Arzola C, Davies S, Rofaeel A, Carvalho JC (2007) Ultrasound using the transverse approach to the lumbar spine provides reliable landmarks for labor epidurals. *Anesthesia and Analgesia* **104:** 1188–92

Cedergren MI (2004) Maternal morbid obesity and the risk of adverse pregnancy outcome. *Obstetrics and Gynecology* **103:** 219–24

CEMACH (2007) The Confidential Enquiry into Maternal and Child Health. Saving Mothers' Lives. 2003–2005

Collins JS, Lemmens HJ, Brodsky JB, Brock-Utne JG, Levitan RM (2004) Laryngoscopy and morbid obesity: a comparison of the 'sniff' and 'ramped' positions. *Obesity Surgery* **14:** 1171–5

Cooper GM, McClure JH (2005) Anaesthesia. In: The Confidential Enquiry into Maternal and Child Health (CEMACH). Why Mothers Die. 2000–2002

Hawthorne L, Wilson R, Lyons G, Dresner M (1996), Failed intubation revisited: 17 year experience in a teaching maternity unit. *British Journal of Anaesthesia* **76:** 595–600

Hodgkinson R, Husain FJ (1980) Caesarean section associated with gross obesity. *British Journal of Anaesthesia* **52:** 919–23

Hood DD, Dewan DM (1993) Anesthetic and obstetric outcome in morbidly obese parturients. *Anesthesiology* **199**(79): 1210–8

Juvin P, Lavaut E, Dupont H, Lefevre P (2003) Difficult tracheal intubation is more common in obese than lean patients. *Anesthesia and Analgesia* **97:** 595–600

McClelland S, Bogod D, Hardman J (2009) Pre-oxygenation and apnoea in pregnancy: changes during labour and with obstetric morbidity in a computational simulation. *Anaesthesia* **64**(4): 1365–2044

McCrae AF (2009) Morbidly obese patients should not be anaesthetised by trainees without supervision. *International Journal of Obstetric Anesthesia* **18:** 373–6

Mhyre J (2007) A Series of Anesthesia-Related Maternal Deaths in Michigan, 1985-2003. *Obstetrical & Gynecological Survey* **62**(10): 645–6

Perlow JH, Morgan MA (1994) Massive maternal obesity and perioperative cesarean morbidity. *American Journal of Obstetrics and Gynecology* **170:** 560–5

Saravanakumar K, Rao SG, Cooper GM (2006) Obesity and obstetric anaesthesia, *Anaesthesia* **61:** 36–48

Tsueda K, Debrand M, Zeok SS, Wright BD, Griffin WO (1979) Obesity supine death syndrome: reports of two morbidly obese patients. *Anesthesia and Analgesia* **58:** 345–7

Whitty RJ, Maxwell CV, Carvalho JCA (2006) Complications of neuraxial anesthesia in an extreme morbidly obese patient for cesarean section. *International Journal of Obstetric Anesthesia* **16:** 139–44

Chapter 9

Potential Problems for the Baby of the Obese Mother

Laura de Rooy and Jane Hawdon

Maternal obesity and the baby – what to expect

The risks to mothers during and after a pregnancy complicated by obesity have been covered extensively in this book. It is also important to consider the risks to the fetus and baby so that management of the mother and baby can be planned accordingly.

Obesity is often a co-morbidity with other risk factors for poor fetal and neonatal outcome e.g. diabetes, smoking, psychosocial concerns. Therefore these conditions must also be looked for and managed according to best practice.

However there is growing evidence for a link between maternal obesity and poor pregnancy outcomes. In a Danish study by Kristensen et al (2005), maternal obesity (BMI >30 kg/m2) was associated with a more than doubled risk of stillbirth and neonatal death (odds ratio (OR) = 2.8, 95% confidence interval (CI): 1.5-5.3; and odds ratio = 2.6, 95% CI: 1.2-5.8). A meta-analysis of 9 studies, conducted by Chu et al (2007), demonstrated a two fold increase in the stillbirth rate among obese women.

In the UK, data from the Confidential Enquiry into Maternal and Child Health (CEMACH) (2006) shows that of the women who had a stillbirth and a recorded BMI, 26% were obese (BMI >30 kg/m2) and for neonatal deaths, 22% were obese (*Table 9.1*). Without national denominator data no definitive conclusions can be drawn, but these numbers do indicate that obese women were overrepresented in pregnancies complicated by a perinatal loss. The CEMACH has commenced work on an important project, due to report in 2011, which will allow the demographics and outcomes for pregnant women with obesity in the UK to be more closely defined (CEMACH 2008).

There is a continuum of risk: as BMI increases, so the risks of fetal demise or neonatal death increase (Thompson et al 2008). In addition, gestational weight gain impacts upon maternal and infant outcomes. Women with a normal prepregnancy BMI who gained excessive weight in pregnancy showed an increased rate of gestational hypertension, augmentation of labour, and birth weight >4000grams (Crane et al 2009).

Table 9.1 Percentage distribution of stillbirths, perinatal and neonatal deaths by mother's BMI: England, Wales and Northern ireland: 2006

Body Mass Index	Still births Number	%	Perinatal deaths Number	%	Neonatal deaths Number	%
Total	3,493		5,075		2,070	
<18.5	80	2.7	123	3.0	58	3.6
18.5-24.9	1,273	43.5	1,820	43.5	724	45.0
25-29.9	810	27.7	1,197	28.6	471	29.3
30+	761	26.0	1,040	24.9	356	22.1
Missing	569		891		461	

Note 1: Percentages are calculated removing missing and not known
Note 2: Second or subsequent deaths from pregnancies with multiple losses excluded from this table

The biomechanisms for fetal/neonatal death in association with maternal obesity are poorly understood. Chen et al (2009) reported that neonatal death in pregnancies complicated by maternal obesity resulted from pregnancy complications or disorders relating to short gestations and unspecified low birth weight. While some work has shown that the important co-morbities present in the obese pregnancy may explain some of the excess risk of neonatal death (Naeye 1990), this is not a universal finding (Kristensen 2005). Research on animals showed placental structural and functional changes in obese baboons (Farley et al 2009). Kristensen (2005) hypothesised that the observed hyperlipidaemia in obesity might lead to a reduction of thromboxane production with an increased risk of placental thrombosis and decreased placental perfusion and so would help explain the observed increased risk of stillbirth in obese women caused by feto-placental dysfunction.

Birth defects and maternal obesity

Both maternal diabetes and maternal obesity is associated with fetal malformations. The CEMACH study found almost double the rate of congenital anomalies in babies born to diabetic mothers compared to the general population (CEMACH 2007). Most of this increase was accounted for by a three fold increase in the rate of neural tube and congenital heart defects. There is also a documented association between maternal obesity and birth defects (Callaway et al 1996) (*Table 9.2*).

It is difficult to dissect out the relative contributions of obesity and

Table 9.2 Birth defects and maternal obesity

	OR (95% CI)	Source
Birth defects (maternal BMI 30.01- 40 kg/m2)	1.58 (1.02-2.46)	Callaway et al
Birth defects (maternal BMI > 40 kg/m2)	3.41 (1.67-6.94)	

diabetes upon the congenital abnormality rate. A meta-analysis conducted by Stothard et al (2009) found a small increase in the risk of neural tube defects, spina bifida, cardiovascular anomalies, septal anomalies, cleft palate, anorectal atresia, hydrocephaly and limb reduction anomalies among obese mothers. The risk of gastroschisis was significantly reduced. This increase in risk remained even when women with pregestational diabetes were excluded from the analysis. This suggests that most of the reported risk of increased fetal malformations associated with maternal obesity may be mediated by maternal diabetes either pre-dating pregnancy or developed during pregnancy with obesity contributing a smaller amount of direct risk.

The aetiologies for fetal malformations in pregnancy complicated by obesity would therefore be expected to overlap those for women with diabetes in pregnancy. Considerable experimental animal work has been done to help elucidate the pathway of fetal malformation in the diabetic pregnancy. Hyperglycaemia may act as a teratogen, as reactive oxidant species are increased in the hyperglycaemic state. Morgan et al (2008) demonstrated that neural crest cells, vital for the development of cardiac structures, are particularly vulnerable to oxidant stress, as they have low endogenous antioxidant capacity. Neural crest cell apoptosis has been demonstrated in mouse embryos of diabetic mothers subjected to oxidative stress on day 7.5 of gestation. Eriksson et al (1993) found that the addition of a radical scavenging enzyme, superoxide dismutase (SOD), in cultured rat embryos protected against the teratogenic effects of hyperglycaemia.

The concept of fuel-mediated teratogenesis postulated by Norbert Freinkel and colleagues (1986) describes the adverse effects upon the fetus developing in an adverse metabolic milieu. In his work, developing rat embryos exposed to either hyperglycaemia or hyperketonaemia, or both, displayed a significantly higher rate of malformations compared to control groups. The insult to the fetus resulting from an adverse stimulus varies at different times of gestation according to the fetus' developmental timetable. Hyperglycaemia and hyperaminoacidemia in the third trimester produce adverse effects with enhanced development of the fetal islets of Langerhans with hypertrophy of the endocrine pancreas and hyperplasia of β cells. This in turn gives rise to the development of macrosomia and postnatal hypoglycaemia.

What other pathways besides those also active in the diabetic pregnancy mediate birth defects in pregnancies in obese women? Obese women are at an increased risk of having a pregnancy affected by a neural tube defect and more particularly spina bifida (Shaw et al 1996). Moreover, this risk does not appear to be modified by folic acid fortification of foodstuffs (Mojtabai 2004). One study compared serum folate levels in obese and non-obese women of childbearing age, and found lower levels in the obese group. It was estimated that women with a BMI >30 kg/m2 needed an additional 350 mcg/day of folic acid to achieve the same serum levels as women in the <20 kg/m2 BMI category. It was postulated that lower serum folate levels were a possible mechanism linking higher maternal BMI's to an increased risk of neural tube defects in their offspring (Ray et al 2005).

Chittaranjan Yajnik (2009) as part of his work on the Pune Maternal Nutrition Study, advances the interesting concept of nutrient–mediated teratogenesis, supplementing Freinkel's idea of fuel-mediated teratogenesis. Yajnik's concept builds on the idea of intra-uterine programming developed by Barker (1997). In nutrient-mediated teratogenesis, an imbalance or deficiency in certain micro-nutrients is postulated to have a profound 'programming' effect upon the developing fetus. In the Pune study, it was found that maternal vitamin B12 deficiency, together with high maternal folate levels, predicted childhood adiposity and insulin resistance at 6 years of age. Obesity may, of course, be related to overnutrition of fat and carbohydrate, but this should not be taken to imply balanced nutrition. In fact, obesity is more prevalent amongst lower socio-economic groups where poor balance of nutrition is also more commonly noted.

The Barker hypothesis: fetal programming in diabetic and obese pregnancies

The Barker hypothesis, supported by a wealth of animal and human epidemiological work, postulates that sub-optimal nutritional conditions in utero program the metabolic adaptation of the fetus so that it is prepared for survival in a resource poor environment, the so-called 'thrifty phenotype' (Hales and Barker 2001). Such an infant, exposed to a postnatal environment with plentiful nutrition will be more likely to develop components of the metabolic syndrome (obesity, hypertension, glucose intolerance and dyslipidaemia) in later life. In diabetic pregnancies, an oversupply of nutrients throughout pregnancy may also program the fetus for future abnormal metabolism; studies in the Pima Indian community showed that children born to mothers who had diabetes while pregnant (intra-uterine exposure) had a greatly increased risk of diabetes themselves compared to children whose mothers developed diabetes after pregnancy (genetic predisposition) (Dabelea et al 2000). Thus, diabetes in pregnancy appears to be a powerful factor in the propagation of diabetes between the generations, and may be more important than genetic factors.

There may be some overlap between the in-utero programming of babies born to diabetic and obese mothers, although at present the mechanism underlying this later process is poorly elucidated. Work from Boney et al (2005) showed that children exposed to maternal obesity in pregnancy were at increased risk of developing metabolic syndrome later in childhood, as were the large-for-gestational age offspring of mothers with diabetes.

Neonatal morbidity

High maternal weight is associated with an increase in neonatal morbidity such as fetal macrosomia, shoulder dystocia, preterm delivery, admission to neonatal intensive care, and jaundice (Callaway et al 2006; Leddy et al 2008).

Fetal macrosomia

Fetal macrosomia can only be accurately diagnosed after delivery, as the antenatal estimation of fetal weight is notoriously unreliable in later gestation and at higher fetal weights. Definitions of macrosomia differ in the literature, with some studies using a cut-off of 4000 grams, and others a cut-off of 4500 grams. However, as morbidity rises sharply after 4500 grams (Zhang et al 2008), this may be the more clinically relevant threshold value. The incidence for birth weight above 4500 grams is approximately 1.5% in the United States. Maternal risk factors for fetal macrosomia include: obesity, excessive weight gain in pregnancy, diabetes in pregnancy, and a history of delivering a macrosomic infant. A rising incidence of obesity amongst women of childbearing age would suggest that the problem of the baby that is too large is here to stay *(Table 9.3)*.

Shoulder dystocia

Although rare (with an incidence of between 0.5-1.5% of all deliveries), shoulder dystocia is a serious obstetric emergency, and one where fetal hypoxaemia may result unless speedily resolved. The risk of shoulder dystocia is not confined to the larger baby: 50% of shoulder dystocia cases occur in babies weighing <4000 grams. However the risk of shoulder

Table 9.3 Adverse neonatal outcomes associated with maternal obesity

	OR (95% CI)	Source
Admission to neonatal intensive care (maternal BMI > 40 kg/m2)	2.77(1.81-4.25)	Callaway et al (2006)
Premature delivery (< 34 weeks gestation, maternal BMI > 40 kg/m2)	2.13 (1.13-4.01)	
Jaundice (maternal BMI > 40 kg/m2)	1.44 (1.09-1.89)	
Macrosomia (Birth weight > 4500grams)	2.0 (1.4-3.0)	Leddy et al (2008)
Shoulder dystocia	3.6 (2.1-6.3)	

dystocia does increase with larger birth weights, complicating 9.2-24% of vaginal deliveries of babies >4500 grams (Pundir and Sinha 2009). The relative disproportion of head and trunk size may be critical in the association of macrosomia and shoulder dystocia. Until about 36 weeks, the fetal head is larger than the trunk. Thereafter, the size of the trunk and shoulders increases relative to the head. This is most marked in diabetic pregnancies and at earlier gestations, as here there is excess supply of glucose to the fetus, resulting in excess adiposity, but is also seen in pregnancies of prolonged gestation. It is likely that this disproportion pervades in macrosomic babies of pregnant women with obesity (Lerner 2004). Other birth injuries, such as brachial plexus injury and clavicular fracture are also more common in the macrosomic infant, especially where there is shoulder dystocia. In a study from Raio et al (2003) the rate of brachial plexus injury increases steadily from 0.8% in babies in the 4500-4599 weight catergory, to 2.86% in babies weighing more than 5000 grams.

Breastfeeding

Despite the recognised benefits for both mother and child, breastfeeding rates vary enormously across the world, with low initiation rates reported in the USA (70.1%) and UK (69%), and far higher rates reported in Denmark

(98%) and other Scandanavian countries. In addition, rates of continued breastfeeding are low in countries such as the UK, with only 21% of mothers continuing to breastfeed at 4-5 months (La Leche League 2003). Numerous factors influence a women's decision to breastfeed her baby. The various associations with breastfeeding behaviour have been the subject of intensive study in those countries with low rates – with the objective that an understanding of the factors inhibiting the establishment of successful breastfeeding will allow the effective targeting of health interventions. Generally, mothers who breastfeed are older, wealthier and have higher levels of education than those who do not.

Most large studies show that obese women plan to breastfeed for a shorter period, and are less likely to initiate and sustain breastfeeding. Amir and Donath (2007) in their review of maternal obesity, breastfeeding intention, initiation and duration, showed that the odds ratio of not initiating breastfeeding was 1.19-2.17 for overweight women compared to normal weight women, and 1.38-3.09 for obese women. Li et al (2003) in their American study of maternal obesity and breastfeeding practices adjusted their findings for 10 possible confounding variables such as socio-economic status, maternal education, ethnicity and baby's birth weight and found that both maternal BMI before pregnancy and gestational weight gain independently affected the continuation of breastfeeding. Women who were obese before pregnancy breast fed two weeks less than did women who were of normal weigh; women who gained either less than, or more than, the recommended weight during pregnancy breast fed one week less than did those who gained the recommended weight.

The independent effect of maternal obesity upon breast feeding behaviour may be small on an individual basis, but important from a population perspective, especially as it may assist in targetting this group of mothers for breastfeeding support interventions.

The mechanisms for the observed association between maternal obesity and poor breastfeeding behaviour are multiple and may include biological, social and cultural factors. There is some animal based evidence for reduced and delayed lactation in obesity (Flint et al 2005; Rasmussen 1998). Several studies have investigated delayed lactogenesis II (the milk 'coming in') in obese women (Rasmussen and Kjolhede 2004). While there is some evidence for reduced levels of prolactin in response to suckling in lactating obese women, there is no evidence that this is mediated by abnormally high progesterone levels. Size and shape of the breast in mothers with obesity may make it more difficult to achieve a good latch. Women with obesity are more likely to have an assisted delivery or caesarean and so will be less mobile after delivery. This means they may experience physical barriers to breastfeeding, especially if optimal lactation support is not in place (Jevitt et al 2007). Social factors are less easily defined: being overweight or having larger breasts may make it more difficult to breastfeed discreetly and thus women may be deterred by modesty, as suggested by Amir and Donath's review of this subject.

While breastfeeding remains the gold standard for all infant feeding, there are specific benefits for both mothers and babies where there is maternal obesity or overweight. A study from Denmark (where breastfeeding rates are high) showed that breastfeeding was associated with reduced post partum weight retention at six months in a dose-dependent fashion across the spectrum of prepregnancy BMI's (Baker et al 2007). In the longer term, there is evidence to suggest that an increased duration of lactation is associated with lower prevalence of hypertension, diabetes, hyperlipidaemia and cardiovascular disease in postmenopausal women (Schwarz et al 2009). Other long term benefits include a reduction in the risk of breast cancer and a possible reduced risk of ovarian cancer. A review written by Horta et al and published by the World Health Organisation in 2008 showed that for babies, breastfeeding confers a reduced risk of obesity and type 1 diabetes, with some evidence for a reduction in the risk of type 2 diabetes. Two large population studies published after this review showed no protective effect of breastfeeding on the development of obesity at five years of age (Sweden: Huus et al 2008) or at 11 years of age (Brazil: Neutzling et al 2009). However, there is good evidence to suggest that growth is different for breastfed infants in the first year, with a lower trajectory from 6 months onwards: the World Health Organisation have recently published their new growth charts, which use exclusively breastfed infants as the norm. A further study from Germany (Kalies et al, 2005) showed a protective effect of exclusive breastfeeding for six months on elevated weight gain at two years of age. Breastfeeding may therefore have a maximal impact on early weight gain, with other factors coming into play as the child grows older. As there is evidence to suggest that infants born to obese mothers may have up to three times the risk of developing obesity later in life compared to children born to mothers of a normal weight (Al-Qaoud and Prakash 2009), the positive effect of breastfeeding is even more important in this group of infants.

Neonatal hypoglycaemia

There is some support for the notion that the large-for-gestational age (LGA) infant is at risk of neonatal hypoglycaemia even in the absence of overt maternal diabetes (Schaefer-Graf et al 2002; Araz and Araz 2006) and so should be screened for hypoglycaemia, in the same way that such screening is performed for the infant of the diabetic mother. However, Schaeffer-Graf's work demonstrates that hypoglycaemia in the LGA population is most strongly associated with elevated maternal one and two hour oral glucose tolerance tests rather than birth weight. In addition, the major burden (>85%) of hypoglycaemia (here defined as a blood glucose level of <30 mg/dl or 1.67 mmol/l) fell within the first five postnatal hours. There is good evidence for a normal decline in blood glucose values to less than 2 mmol/l in this time window (Srinivasan et al 1986). A retrospective analysis of 457 infant records from Van Howe and Storms (2008) found no evidence that higher birth weight increases the risk for hypoglycaemia. A smaller study from de Rooy and Hawdon (1992) indicated that while LGA babies did have documented low blood glucose values (as do babies of normal birth weight), this was offset by a normal ketone body response as seen in appropriate-for-gestational age (AGA) infants. Ketone bodies are important in neonatal metabolic adaptation in that they provide an alternative source of energy to the brain besides glucose.

Work from Brand et al (2005) provide further reassurance in demonstrating that transient, mild hypoglycaemia (defined as <2.2mmol/l at 1 hour after birth, and <2.5 mmol/l thereafter) in healthy term LGA infants does not appear to be harmful to psychomotor development at four years of age. It would seem, based on present evidence, that routine screening for hypoglycaemia is not necessary for all LGA infants, unless significant co-morbidities, such as an abnormal maternal glucose tolerance test or prematurity co-exists.

Conclusion

In this chapter we have attempted to elucidate some of the risks to the fetus and baby of the mother with obesity. While such risks are important from a population perspective, it should be remembered that the risk to an individual may still be small – double or treble the risk of a rare event is still, after all, a rare event. Knowledge of the risks pertaining to the obese pregnancy should be used to inform health professionals and help them to provide and tailor services for women with increased risks. More importantly perhaps, such knowledge should be used to empower women to make healthy lifestyle choices for themselves and their families.

References

Al-Qaoud N, Prakash P (2009)Can breastfeeding and its duration determine the overweight status of Kuwaiti children at the age of 3-6 years? Eur J Clin Nutr. 63 (8):1041-3

Amir LH, Donath SM (2007) A systematic review of maternal obesity and breastfeeding intention and duration. *BMC Pregnancy Childbirth* **7**:9

Araz N, Araz M (2006) Frequency of neonatal hypoglycaemia in large for gestational age infants of non-diabetic mothers in a community maternity hospital Acta Medica 49(4):237-9.

Baker JL, Michaelsen KF, Sorenson TIA et al (2007) High prepregnant bodymass index is associated with early termination of full and any breastfeeding in Danish women. *American journal of Clinical Nutrition* **86**(2); 404-11

Barker DJP (1997) Maternal Nutrition, Fetal Nutrition, and Disease in Later Life. *Nutrition* **13**(9): 807-13

Boney CM, Verma A, Tucker R et al (2005) Metabolic Syndrome in Childhood: Association with birth weight, maternal obesity, and gestational diabetes mellitus. *Pediatr* **115**(3): e290-96

Brand PL, Molenaar NL, Kaaijk C et al (2005) Neurodevelopmental outcome of hypoglycaemia in healthy, large for gestational age, term newborns. Arch Dis Child. 90 (1):78-81.

Callaway LK, Prins JB, Chang AM et al.(2006) The prevalence and impact of overweight and obesity in an Australian Obstetric population. *MJA* **184**(2):56-9

Crane JM, White J, Murphy P et al (2009) The Effects of gestational weight gain by body mass index on maternal and neonatal outcomes. *J Obstet Gynaecol Can* **31**(1):28-35.

Confidential Enquiry into Maternal and Child Health (2006) *Perinatal mortality 2006: England, Wales and Northern Ireland*. CEMACH: London, 2008.

Confidential Enquiry into Maternal and Child Health (2007) *Diabetes in Pregnancy: Are we providing the best care? Findings of a National Enquiry:* England, Wales and Northern Ireland. CEMACH: London

Confidential Enquiry into Maternal and Child Health (2008) http://www.cemach.org.uk/ Programmes/Maternal-and-Perinatal/Maternal-Obesity.aspx

Chu SY, Kim SY, Lau J et al (2007) Maternal obesity and risk of stillbirth: a meta analysis. *Am J Obstet Gynecol* **197**(3): 223-8

Dabelea D, Knowler WC, Pettitt DJ (2000) Effect of diabetes in pregnancy on offspring: follow-up research in the Pima Indians. *J Matern Fetal Med* **9**(1):83-8

Eriksson UJ, Borg LA (1993) Diabetes and embryonic malformations. Role of substrate-induced free-oxygen radical production for dysmorphogenesis in cultured rat embryos. *Diabetes* **42**: 411-19.

Farley D, Tejero ME, Comuzzie AG et al (2009) Feto-placental Adaptations to Maternal Obesity in the baboon. Placenta 30 (9):752-760

Flint DJ, Travers MT, Barber MC et al (2005) Diet-induced obesity impairs mammary development and lactogensesis in murine mammary glands. *Am J Physiol Endocrinol Metab* **288**(6):E1179-87. Epub 2005 Jan 25.

Freinkel N, Cockcroft D, Lewis N (1986) The 1986 McCollum award lecture. Fuel-mediated teratogenesis during early organogenesis: the effects of increased concentrations of glucose, ketones or somatomedin inhibitor during rat embryo culture. *American Journal of Clinical Nutrition*.

Hales NC, Barker DJP (2001) The thrifty phenotype hypothesis. *British Medical Bulletin* **60**:5-20

Horta BL, Bahl R, Martines JC, Victora CG (2007) *Evidence of long-term effects of breastfeeding. Systematic reviews and meta-analyses*. World Health Organisation

Huus K, Ludvigsson JF, Enskär K, Ludvigsson J (2008) Exclusive breastfeeding of Swedish children and its possible influence on the development of obesity : a prospective cohort study. BMC Pediatr. 8:42

Jevitt C, Hernandez I, Groër M (2007) Lactation complicated by overweight and obesity: supporting the mother and newborn. *J Midwifery Womens Health* **52**(6):606-13

Kalies H, Heinrich J, Borte N, LISA Study Group (2005) *Eur J Med Res* **10**(1): 36-42

Kristensen J, Vestergaard M, Wisborg K et al (2005) Pre-pregnancy weight and the risk of stillbirth and neonatal death . *BJOG* **112**(4): 403-8

La Leche League International (2003) http://www.llli.org/cbi/bfstats03.html

Leddy MA, Power ML, Schulkin J (2008) The impact of Maternal Obesity on Maternal and Fetal Health. *Reviews in Obsterics and Gynecology* **1**(4)

Lerner, H.(2004) http://www.shoulderdystociainfo.com

Li R, Jewell S, Grummer-Strawn L (2003) Maternal Obesity and breastfeeding practices. Am J Clin Nutr. 77(4):931-936.

Morgan SC, Relaix F, Sandell LL et al (2008) Oxidative stress during diabetic pregnancy disrupts cardiac neural crest migration and causes outflow defects. *Birth Defects Res A Clin Mol Teratol* **70**:927-38

Mojtabai R (2004) Body mass index and serum folate in childbearing age women. *European journal of Epidemiology* **19**:1029-36

Naeye RL (1990) Maternal Body weight and pregnancy outcome. Am J Clin Nutr. 52 (2):273-9.

Neutzling MB, Hallal PR, Araujo CL et al (2009) Infant feeding and onbesity at 11 years: Propsective birth cohort study. *Int J Pediatr Obes*.**7**:1-7.

Pundir J, Sinha P (2009) Non-diabetic macrosomia:an obstetric dilemma. *J Obstet Gynecol* **29**(3):200-5.

Raio L, Ghezzi F, Di Naro E (2003) Perinatal outcome of fetuses with a birth weight greater than 4500 g: an analysis of 3356 cases. *Eur J Obstet Gynecol Reprod Biol*.**109**(2): 160-5.

Rasmussen (1998): Rasmussen KM (1998) Effect of under- and overnutrition on lactation in laboratory rats. J Nutr. 128 (2 Suppl): 390S-393S.

Ray JG, Wyatt PR, Vermeulen MJ et al (2005) Greater maternal weight and the ongoing risk of neural tube defects after folic acid flour fortification. *Obstet Gynecol* **105**(2):261-5.

Schwarz EB, Ray RM, Stuebe AM et al (2009) Duration of lactation and risk factors for maternal cardiovascular disease. *Obstet Gynecol* **113**(5):972-3.

Stothard KJ, Tennant PW, Bell R et al (2009) Maternal overweight and obesity and the risk of congenital anomalies: a systematic review and meta-analysis. *JAMA* **301**(6):636-50.

Shaw GM, Velie EM, Schaffer D (1996) Risk of neural tube defect-affected pregnancies amongst obese women. *JAMA* **275**:1093-1096.

Srinivasan G, Pildes RS, Cattamanchi G et al (1986) Plasma glucose values in normal neonates: a new look. J Pediatr 109 (1):114-7.

Thompson DR, Clark CL, Wood B et al (2008) Maternal Obesity and risk of infant death based on Florida birth records for 2004. *Public Health Rep* **123**(4): 487-93

Yajnik CS (2009) Nutrient-mediated teratogenesis and fuel-mediated teratogenesis: two pathways of intrauterine programming of diabetes. *Int J Gynaecol Obstet* **104** Suppl 1: 1:S27-31

Zhang X, Decker A, Platt RW et al (2008) How big is too big? The perinatal consequences of fetal macrosomia. *Am J Obstet Gynecol* **198**(5):517.e10-6.

Chapter 10

Effective Postnatal Care

Debra Bick

Introduction

"...The priority for modern maternity services is to provide a choice of safe, high quality maternity care for all women and their partners. This is to enable pregnancy and birth to be as safe and satisfying as possible for both mother and baby and to support new parents to have a confident start to family life. For some, especially the more vulnerable and disadvantaged, the outcomes are unacceptable. Some women are up to 20 times more likely to die from a pregnancy related complication than other women and infant mortality rates are higher in more deprived areas of the country and in more vulnerable or disadvantaged groups..."
　　　Maternity Matters (Department of Health 2007)

Midwifery care of women in the immediate hours and days following birth became a statutory requirement in the early 20th century. The midwife's role included daily physical observations and examinations of a woman's temperature, pulse, assessment of her lochia and uterine involution. The aim of this proscriptive content of care was to detect post partum haemorrhage (PPH) and puerperal sepsis, the main causes of maternal mortality at the time the first Midwives Act was passed in 1902. The majority of midwifery contacts then took place in a woman's home with the number and timing of home visits regulated for all women and specified in the midwives rules (Central Midwives Board 1905). A woman had to be visited by a midwife twice a day for the first three days and then daily until day ten.

　　The introduction of the statutory provision of midwifery postnatal care as required by the 1902 Midwives Act and the predetermined pattern of visits set out in the midwives rules was established in reaction to the then high maternal mortality rate, which did not decline until around the time of the Second World War, when the rate declined steeply as a consequence of several factors, including better public health, development of antibiotics and introduction of obstetric flying squads. Relatively little revision to the content and timing of midwifery postnatal care has occurred since 1905 and midwifery postnatal care continues to be a statutory requirement in the UK. This is despite the fact that the majority of women now give birth in the hospital; health and social needs have dramatically changed; and midwives have been able to make 'selective' rather than daily postnatal domiciliary visits for 10 days since 1986.

Research undertaken since the 1990's has highlighted widespread and persistent maternal health problems after giving birth, many of which persist well beyond the 6–8 week postnatal period (MacArthur et al 1991; Glazener et al 1995). Of note was that women did not report problems to their midwives and the current model of postnatal care did not identify them as it focused instead on a traditional content of care which included physical observations and examinations such as uterine involution and vaginal loss.

Clearly the routine provision of care was not meeting the needs of women, and it has also become evident that the health profile of women who give birth in the UK has changed dramatically during the last decade. Today, the general health of women who become pregnant is poorer for a number of reasons which reflect at a micro level an individual's lifestyle choices, and at a macro level, the need to escape conflict or political persecution. For example women from some parts of the world who seek refuge or asylum in the UK may have their health comprised by TB, female genital cutting and consequences of sustained poor nutrition. In developed countries, there is an increasing trend for women to delay childbirth and an epidemic of obesity, which has a significant impact on pregnancy and longer-term health outcomes (Lewis 2007). While the focus of this chapter is the postnatal care of women who are obese (defined as a Body Mass Index (BMI) of ≥30), it is important to remember that all women require effective postnatal care and other factors such as a woman's ethnicity, or her exposure to a myriad of social problems, including domestic violence, can also lead to poorer pregnancy outcomes (Mander and Smith 2008; Knight et al 2009).

Background

Before considering what effective postnatal care could mean in terms of planning, content and resource use, it is important to consider how being obese during pregnancy can impact on the health of a woman and her baby. The most recent triennial report of maternal deaths in the UK (Lewis 2007) highlighted in stark terms why obesity is such a crucial public health issue:

"More than half of all the women who died from Direct or Indirect causes, for whom information was available, were either overweight or obese. More than 15% of all women who died from Direct or Indirect causes were morbidly or super morbidly obese."

Furthermore, Lewis (2007) reported that maternal obesity is one of the greatest and growing overall threats to the childbearing population of the UK. Obesity was a common factor among women who died during 2003–2005 from thromboembolism, sepsis and cardiac disease. For example, 14 of 31 women with a known BMI who died following a thromboembolic event were obese. For each woman who died as a direct or indirect consequence of pregnancy where obesity was a contributing factor, it is likely that other women who experienced an adverse obstetric event, such as a post-partum haemorrhage, were saved due to effective and prompt emergency care.

Obesity does not only impact the health of the woman. Recent research has considered the impact on the baby in utero and during the early years of life. An obese woman has an increased risk of restricted fetal growth during her first pregnancy (Rajasingham et al 2009), a higher risk of structural fetal anomalies (Stothard et al 2009) and her child is at higher risk of developing diabetes (Leddy et al 2008). The 2005 Confidential Enquiry into Maternal and Child Health (CEMACH) Perinatal Mortality report found that around 30% of mothers who had a stillbirth or neonatal death had a BMI of ≥30. A meta-analysis by Chu et al (2007a) that examined factors associated with stillbirth (six cohort studies and three case control studies were included) found the odds of stillbirth were almost twice as high among obese women compared to women classed as normal weight (OR 2.7, 95% CI 1.59–2.74). Several mechanisms to account for this risk have been proposed, including increased risk of an obese women developing diabetes and hypertensive disorders during pregnancy (Goldenberg et al 2004), utero fetal programming (de Boo and Harding 2006), and inability for an obese woman to feel diminished fetal movements (Fretts et al 2005). The exact relationship between maternal obesity and stillbirth remains unknown and further research is required to assess if it is an independent effect or a consequence of co-morbidity associated with obesity during pregnancy.

The CEMACH 2007 (Lewis 2007) report presented the following as the main risk factors for pregnancy and postnatal complications for an obese woman and her infant.

For the mother, there is an increased risk of:

- Maternal death or severe morbidity
- Cardiac disease
- Spontaneous first trimester and recurrent miscarriage
- Pre eclampsia (PE)
- Gestational diabetes
- Thromboembolism
- Post caesarean wound infection
- Infection from other causes
- Post partum haemorrhage
- Low breast feeding rates.

For her baby, there is an increased risk of:
- Stillbirth and neonatal death
- Congenital abnormalities
- Prematurity.

Those complications which are more likely to be experienced as a maternal postnatal event will be addressed later in this chapter.

The numbers of women of childbearing age who are obese has been steadily increasing during the last decade. National statistics on the prevalence of obesity in pregnant and postnatal women has not been collated in the UK, however CEMACH have launched a national programme on obesity in pregnancy which will include information on the provision of services to obese women, care standards, local and national prevalence figures, pregnancy outcomes and an audit of clinical care (Lewis 2007). National data on women who have a BMI of ≥35 will be recorded. The decision to use this measure was based on the view that recommendations for care would be easier to implement and change in practice could be more substantial with respect to improved outcomes (CEMACH 2009).

Data on severe maternal morbidity in pregnant and postnatal women have also not been routinely collated in England. An ongoing audit of severe morbidity has taken place in Scotland since 2001(Penney et al 2007) which collected data for 14 categories, ranging from major post partum haemorrhage (PPH), pulmonary oedema, cardiac arrest and massive pulmonary embolism. Rates of events per 1,000 women rose from 4.6 in 2004 to 6.1 in 2005, an increase greater than that expected by chance. The UK Obstetric Surveillance System (UKOSS) survey which is a joint initiative between the National Perinatal Epidemiology Unit and the Royal College of Obstetricians and Gynaecologists, was launched in 2005 to collate data on severe maternal morbidity on a national population basis (Knight et al 2008). Data were collated on a range of rare conditions in pregnancy (those with an estimated incidence of fewer than one in 2000 births) which can adversely affect the outcome for a woman and/or her baby, including antenatal stroke, myocardial infarction and extreme obesity (classed as a BMI of ≥50). Nominated staff at each of the 227 consultant led obstetric units in the UK were asked to provide details of any cases of the conditions under surveillance during the previous month. Case definition for extreme obesity included women who weighed 140kg or more at any time during pregnancy, had a BMI of ≥50, or who were expected to fulfil these two criteria but whose weight exceeded the hospital scales. Preliminary data collected between March 2007 and September 2008 suggests extreme obesity affects one in 1000 women, and that they experience significantly more pregnancy, birth and postnatal complications than comparison women identified as the woman delivering immediately before the case in the same hospital.

Implications of obesity for maternal postnatal health outcomes

It is clear that the numbers of women in the UK who are obese when they become pregnant is increasing and this has implications for their own, and for their baby's, immediate and longer-term health. How or when to deal with this issue is less clear. The implications of obesity for a woman's postnatal health should be a matter of concern for all relevant clinicians as it could affect the content of care and frequency of contact she may require as well as provide an opportunity to influence her future health behaviour. The priorities for practice should include planning postnatal care during pregnancy to prevent and minimise potential post birth complications and assist the woman and her baby to achieve the best possible outcome. This is especially important if the woman has other risk factors, such as being an older mother. Antenatal planning could also have implications for mode of birth, which in itself will influence morbidity outcomes and the level of care a woman will require. Nevertheless, with anecdotal evidence of the relatively low priority now accorded to postnatal care, midwives, managers, service providers and commissioners need to be aware of the challenges for practice and why effective postnatal care could make a difference.

The following section highlights some of the health risks an obese woman may experience during the postnatal period. Much of the data reported are from retrospective studies which may be subject to bias due to incomplete data collection, although studies consistently demonstrate the complexity of health issues faced by an obese woman.

Post wound and other infections

The most recent data on birth outcomes in England during 2007-2008 showed a small increase in the number of births by caesarean section (CS); 24.6% of women gave birth by CS, a 0.3 percentage point increase from the previous year (The Information Centre 2009). Obese women are more likely to have complicated pregnancies which require medical intervention, with the rate of successful vaginal birth decreasing as maternal BMI increases (Leddy et al 2008). A meta-analysis by Chu et al (2007b) on maternal obesity and risk of CS which included 33 studies found that compared to normal weight pregnant women, the odds of a CS birth were:

- 1.46 (95% CI, 1.34-1.60) among overweight
- 2.05 (95% CI 1.86-2.27) among obese
- 2.89 (95% CI 2.28-3.79) among severely obese women.

A CS birth is also associated with a number of potential shorter and longer term maternal health complications including surgical site infection (SSI). Despite the increased number of CS births, the length of time women stay on the inpatient postnatal ward following operative birth has declined (Redshaw et al 2007; The Information Centre 2009) with limited evidence that community midwifery postnatal contacts have been revised to reflect post-surgical, as well as post-birth, needs across the UK.

Surgical site infections may affect the abdominal wound, uterus or endometrium and infection is most likely to become evident in the community. Data on incidence of CS SSI are limited but suggest 10-20% of women develop SSI, based on criteria developed by the US Centers for Disease Control (Horan et al 1992). Prospective data on 715 women who had a CS birth was collected over a 35 week period during 2002-03 from one maternity unit in Scotland by Johnson et al (2006) found 80 women developed a post CS infection. Infection in 57 (71%) of these women was detected following hospital discharge. Obese women had significantly more infections than women with a normal BMI (p=0.028).

Ward and colleagues (2008) collected data from one of the first UK prospective multicentre studies of CS infection outcomes. Data were collected by community midwives on women who had a CS birth at 11 sites in the East Midlands of England for a varying period of between three and 18 months. Of 6297 CS births during the study period, data were available for 5563 women, with a median length of follow-up of 15 days, although there was marked inter-unit variation. A total of 745 SSIs were recorded in 738 (13.3%) of the 5563 women, 488 (65.5%) of which met study definitions of SSI. Risk factors included:

- Maternal BMI (p<0.0001)
- Emergency procedures (p=0.002)
- Spontaneous Rupture of Membranes (SROM) (p=0.01)
- In labour at the time of surgery (p<0.001)
- Duration of procedure (p=0.002)
- Wound closure method (p=0.003).

Maternal BMI was also reported as a risk factor for SSI in the All Wales Annual Report (WHAIP 2007) where CS surveillance was introduced as a mandatory requirement in 2006. Questionnaires were returned by sites for 4540 women, although only 3308 (73%) could be analysed to determine SSI rates. Lack of reliability with respect to completeness of data collection once a woman has been discharged from hospital and lack of application of SSI criteria remain important issues to address given the frequency with which CS is now performed.

The CEMACH (Lewis 2007) reported 22 women died of genital tract sepsis during 2003–2005 including one woman who died following an illegal abortion. The majority of the women who died were overweight; seven women had a BMI greater than 30, three of whom were morbidly obese with a BMI exceeding 35. Ten of the women died from genital tract sepsis following a CS birth. None of the women had any signs of infection until two to seven days after the birth. Given that infection is likely to develop post hospital discharge and that substandard care was noted in 15 cases, the need to ensure effective postnatal care should be accorded a high priority for obese women.

Cardiac disease

Women who are obese are at higher risk of developing cardiac disease during pregnancy. This is not the only risk factor, as those who smoke, have hypertension, diabetes, are older, or have a family history of cardiac disease are also at risk and a woman may present with several risk factors. Cardiac disease was the commonest overall cause of maternal death during the triennium 2003–2005 (Lewis 2007). These deaths were classed as indirect deaths, however the CEMACH enquiry raised concerns about the increase in relative and absolute numbers of women who have ischemic cardiac disease (Lewis 2007). This is a condition more likely to be attributable to a woman's lifestyle choices and as such is potentially preventable. Of 45 maternal deaths from cardiac disease where a BMI was available, 29 women were classed as obese.

There is a dearth of contemporary data with respect to the number of women in the UK who suffer a myocardial infarction (MI) during pregnancy, with the current incidence estimate of 1 in 10000 births based on data collected in 1970 (cited by Knight et al 2008). A retrospective study from California conducted by Ladner and colleagues (2005) which analysed data over a 10 year period to estimate the population incidence and pregnancy outcomes of acute MI found an incidence of 1 in 35700 births, with 41% of events occurring during the six week postnatal period, 38% during pregnancy and 21% during labour. The incidence rate increased over the 10 year study period. The UK Obstetric Survelliance System (UKOSS) has been collating data on pregnancy related MI since 2005, reporting 13 confirmed cases up until January 2008. This was lower than expected and the data collection period has been extended to enable all potential sources of data to be considered (Knight et al 2008).

Pre eclampsia (PE)

Gifford et al (2000) proposed that the hypertensive disorders of pregnancy comprised a spectrum of conditions which could be classified into four categories:

(i)   Gestational hypertension, a rise in blood pressure during the second half of pregnancy

(ii)   PE, usually hypertension with proteinuria (protein in urine) during the second half of pregnancy

(iii)   Chronic hypertension, a rise in blood pressure prior to pregnancy or before 20 weeks' gestation

(iv)   PE superimposed on chronic hypertension.

The precise relationship between PE and pregnancy induced hypertension remains unclear (Bick et al 2008) but symptoms may have a pregnancy or a postnatal onset in a previously normotensive women. One study examined the postnatal duration of hypertension among women who had already presented with pregnancy induced hypertension (PIH) or PE. Ferrazzani et al (1994) studied 269 women with PIH (n=159) or PE (n=110) and monitored their postpartum blood pressure daily after delivery until a diastolic blood pressure of ≤110mmHg was reached. The time taken for this ranged from 0-10 days among the PIH women and from 0-23 days among those with PE. How long it took for women to become 'normotensive' (diastolic ≤80mmHg) however, was not reported.

A number of retrospective studies have shown that a BMI of ≥30 is a risk factor for the development of hypertension and onset of PE in women of all parities (Kerrigan and Kingdon 2009) as well as in women having their first baby (Rajasingham et al 2009). The risk appears to increase further if the woman is morbidly obese (BMI ≥35). Battacharya et al (2007) undertook a retrospective cohort study of women who gave birth to their first baby in Aberdeen between 1976 and 2005. In comparison with women who had a BMI of 20-24.9, morbidly obese women faced the highest risk of PE (OR 7.2, 95% CI 4.7-11.2) and underweight women the lowest (OR 0.6, 95% 0.5-0.7).

The incidence of eclampsia is difficult to ascertain, particularly in postnatal women. An estimated incidence of 2.7 per 10000 maternities in the UK was reported in 2005, a decrease from 4.9 per 10000 maternities in 1992 (Knight et al 2005) which may be attributable to the recommended use of magnesium sulphate to manage these cases. In the most recent CEMACH report (Lewis 2007), 18 women died of eclampsia or PE with one additional woman dying from acute fatty liver of pregnancy. Three women died following discharge from the postnatal ward. A mortality rate of 0.85 per 100000 maternities was similar to those reported in previous triennia.

Thromboembolism

The leading cause of maternal death in the UK remains pulmonary thromboembolism (Lewis 2007). This report showed a total of 41 women died of thrombosis/thromboembolism during 2003–2005, a mortality rate of 1.56 per 100000 maternities. Thirty-three of these women died from pulmonary embolism, 15 of whom died following the birth (seven following a CS birth and eight following a vaginal birth). One encouraging finding was a decline in the death of postpartum pulomonary embolism following CS birth, which may reflect routine use of thromboprophylaxis as recommended in national guidance (RCOG 2007). However, of note was the substandard care of obese women who died following a vaginal birth which in some cases included a lack of thromboprophylaxis.

Post partum haemorrhage (PPH)

Post partum haemorrhage is the single highest cause of maternal mortality and morbidity globally (Roberts et al 2009). The definition of PPH is based on an estimation of blood loss and whether symptoms occurred as:

(i)   Primary: within the first 24 hours of the birth; or
(ii) Secondary: after the first 24 hours and up to six weeks after the birth.

There is no consensus on the exact amount of vaginal blood loss that constitutes a PPH. The World Health Organization (WHO) (2003) defined PPH as 'vaginal bleeding in excess of 500ml after childbirth within or following the first 24 hours'. Precise measurement of blood loss is subject to underestimation and impact on maternal health and wellbeing may also vary according to the individual's haemoglobin level (e.g. a woman with anaemia may be less tolerant of blood loss). Furthermore, studies examining postnatal women's experiences of blood loss imply that there is variability in the normal range of blood loss and reports may only describe most adverse outcomes (Bick et al 2008).

Traditionally, a blood loss greater than 500ml is considered a valid measurement for diagnosing PPH (WHO 2003), while a loss in excess of 1000ml (Stones et al 1993) to 1500ml (Waterstone et al 2001) is proposed to indicate severe or major obstetric haemorrhage. A survey of UK maternity units failed to establish a consistent definition for major PPH but the majority identified blood loss ≥1000ml (46%) or ≥1500ml (36%) as indicators of major PPH (Mousa and Alfirevic 2002). Recent observational studies of morbidity associated with obesity in pregnancy found a higher risk of PPH among obese compared with non obese women, a risk which increased with higher BMI. The retrospective study of effect of BMI on pregnancy outcomes among primiparous women by Bhattacharya et al (2007) found that compared with women who had a BMI of 20–24.9, women who were obese had much greater risk of a PPH (OR 1.5, 95% CI 1.3, 1.7). A smaller retrospective study from South Australia which selected 100 women with normal BMI (BMI 19.1-25), 100 overweight (BMI 25.1-30), 110 obese (BMI 30.1-40) and 60 morbidly obese women (BMI ≥40) were identified with access to complete medical records (Schrauwers and Dekker 2009). Significantly more blood loss was recorded for women who had a BMI of 30.1-40 and ≥40 compared with women who had a BMI of 19.1-25.

Lewis (2007) reported that 14 women died in the UK between 2003–2005 of haemorrhage, with three further cases considered of haemorrhage associated with genital tract trauma and uterine rupture. As CEMACH reports, there has been a significant decline in maternal mortality from PPH during the last 50 years. Nevertheless, as six of the women who died were obese with a BMI of greater than 30, and two were morbidly obese with a BMI of over 35, even with this rare event the risks to the health of obese women is clear. Of more concern was that more than half of the women who died were from ethnic minorities, some of whom were unable to speak English. The number of women who experience an adverse obstetric event such as PPH are increasing, and attention is turning to adverse events as an indicator of the quality of maternity care in high income countries given the rare outcome of maternal death (Roberts et al 2009). This is discussed further in the following section.

Using severe maternal morbidity as an indicator of quality of maternity care

Over recent decades, maternal mortality has been used as an indicator of the quality of the maternity services in the UK. Thankfully, due to advances in public health and clinical management, maternal death in the UK is a rare event. This being the case, there is recognition of the need to use an adverse obstetric event or severe morbidity as a 'complementary marker' of standards of care (Penney et al 2007). Severe morbidity is classed as a health problem that if untreated, could result in the death of the woman. The theory underlying this approach was described by Pattinson et al (2005) as:

> *"the sequence from good health to death in a pregnant woman is a clinical insult, followed by a systemic inflamatory response, organ failure and finally death. A near miss would be those women with organ dysfunction who survive."*

Studies of severe morbidity have tended to be retrospective which may not provide robust, complete data on the factors or outcome related to an event, especially if a woman had been discharged prior to the incident. Studies do however provide useful information on trends over time and can highlight risk factors. In one large population cohort study it was estimated that approximately 1.2% of women experienced severe morbidity. In two thirds of cases this was caused by a massive postpartum haemorrhage, and in one third causes included sepsis, uterine rupture and severe PE (Waterstone et al 2001). Prospective descriptive, cohort or case control studies are important such as those being co-ordinated by UKOSS, however work to capture all adverse events is necessary if the safety and quality of services are to improve. It is important that those who care for obese women are aware that risk factors do not decline at birth and in fact, a woman may be at greater risk of developing complications in the first few hours, days and weeks after giving birth.

In addition to informing how services can be enhanced to improve safety and quality for women at higher risk of complications, information on severe morbidity can also inform how clinical skills can be optimised to detect and manage conditions and the development of appropriate management pathways. Further research could also inform the level of healthcare support and resource a woman may require from pregnancy to beyond the traditional 6–8 week postnatal period (Waterstone et al 2003).

Evidence to support effective postnatal care

Evidence of how postnatal care could be successfully revised to enhance health outcomes is increasing. The large cluster randomised controlled trial (RCT) by MacArthur et al (2002, 2003) showed that midwives who provided community based postnatal care over an extended period of time, informed by use of symptom checklists and evidence based guidance (Bick et al 2008), could make a significant difference to women's shorter and longer-term psychological health. Future work needs to address the postnatal needs of women on the in-patient ward and women with specific health needs, including those associated with obesity. Nevertheless, from the evidence currently available, effective postnatal care could make an important contribution to a woman's future health. This section discusses the evidence currently available to support the planning and content of care to enhance clinical and cost effectiveness with reference to the care of women who are obese.

A framework for effective postnatal care

In 2006 the National Institute for Health and Clinical Excellence (NICE 2006a) published guidelines for the routine postnatal care of healthy women and their babies which presented recommendations for women receiving NHS maternity care in England and Wales. This is part of a suite of guidance for maternity care which includes:

- Antenatal care (NICE 2008a)
- Intrapartum care (NICE 2007a)
- Caesarean section (NICE 2004)
- Diabetes in pregnancy (NICE 2008b)
- Antenatal and postnatal mental health (NICE 2007b)
- Prevention, identification, assessment and management of obesity in adults and children (NICE 2006b)
- Surgical site infection (NICE 2008c)

Health professionals should also be familiar with the Royal College of Obstetricians and Gynaecologists (RCOG) guidance on acute management of thromboembolic disease during pregnancy and the puerperium (RCOG 2007).

All women and their babies will require elements of care as recommended in the NICE postnatal guideline (NICE 2006a), regardless of whether they also require more specialist care. What is important is that for the first time, midwives and other relevant healthcare professionals have guidance on both the timing and content of postnatal contacts, with information to accompany the guidance for women and their partners. The NICE (2006a) guideline recommends that planning for postnatal care should commence antenatally. This is important not just for service providers but for the woman as there is evidence to suggest that women underestimate the impact of birth on their physical and psychological health and have little information on what to expect during the postnatal period (Beake et al 2005). It also means that relevant members of the multi-professional team can be involved in care planning to prevent or minimise postnatal morbidity, for example through advice on prophylaxis to prevent thromboembolism and maintenance of a healthy lifestyle during pregnancy (NICE 2006b).

Physical observations and examinations

There continues to be a dearth of evidence to support how or when midwives should perform routine maternal physical observations and examinations such as assessment of uterine involution, temperature and observation of lochia. Although it is interesting to note that in the trial by MacArthur et al (2003), midwives providing the new model of care reported difficulties with only undertaking physical observations and examinations if indicated, the continued provision of a traditional content of midwifery care cannot be justified if it does not meet the women's needs. Marchant and Garcia (1995) found that despite midwives seeing little value in undertaking traditional observations and examinations at each postnatal contact they continued to do so, reflecting the findings of MacArthur et al (2003). Postnatal care documentation for the most part continues to rely on completion of charts documentating routine observations and examinations, with limited space to record other information or to promote individualised care.

It is now apparent that routine undertaking of physical observations and examinations is not necessary for all women at all contacts. However, it is important that midwives understand the need to ask women at each contact how they are feeling, and follow this up with examination and observation if indicated, based on their clinical judgement or a woman's reporting of signs and symptoms of potential ill health. The NICE (2006a) guidance for core postnatal care recommends that within six hours of the birth a baseline measure of a woman's blood pressure and her first void post birth should be documented, with action to take with respect to both if concern is raised. Furthermore, NICE also recommends that at the first postnatal contact, all women and their partners are offered information on the signs and symptoms of major maternal morbidity including thrombosis, genital tract sepsis, postpartum haemorrhage and PE/eclampsia. If any signs or symptoms of severe ill health are experienced urgent medical attention should be sought. This information is essential for all women given much earlier transfer home from hospital but especially for those who may be at higher risk of adverse outcome, such as women who are obese.

Major morbidity

Midwives and other relevant clinicians must be familiar with signs and symptoms of major postnatal morbidity and retain a high index of suspicion for potential adverse outcome among women who are obese. When planning care for an obese woman, the lead professional co-ordinating care should seek appropriate advice on prophylaxis. In the latest CEMACH report (Lewis 2007), it was noted that midwives and doctors failed to act on signs or symptoms of potential major morbidity and did not appreciate the seriousness of the condition, leading to delays in referral and management. Of note was the failure of midwives, community midwives and doctors to recognise the signs and symptoms of sepsis or to act on findings of routine physical examinations and observations which indicated a potential life threatening illness. As a result of reviewing cases where care was substandard, a recommendation was made by CEMACH (Lewis 2007) that women who are unwell have their physical observations and vital signs monitored using a Modified Early Obstetric Warning Scoring system (MEOWS). The introduction of MEOWS into maternity care requires further consideration. The documentation of signs and symptoms of life threatening illness may not prevent an adverse event, as it is likely to be the action taken by the attending clinician that will make a difference to the outcome. Given the need to tailor care to individual needs which takes into consideration physical and psychological health, research into the effectiveness of the routine use of MEOWS is urgently required.

Commonly experienced postnatal health problems

Research has not been undertaken to identify if women who are obese are at more risk of experiencing commonly experienced health problems after giving birth, such as backache, fatigue, urinary or faecal incontinence, depression and perineal pain. Epidemiological studies have considered the independent effect of factors such as parity, mode of birth, maternal age, obstetric interventions and infant birthweight on maternal morbidity, but BMI has not been routinely included. This may reflect lack of accurate documentation in a woman's maternity record and previous low priority accorded to obesity as a health concern, however this situation is changing (Usha Kiran et al 2005). In a population study from Cardiff (Usha Kiran et al 2005) which included data on over 60 000 births between 1990–1999, adverse outcomes among women having their first baby were compared among women with a BMI of 20–30 and those with a BMI ≥30. With respect to immediate postnatal problems, obese women were more at risk of urinary tract infections and having their baby admitted to the neonatal care unit with feeding difficulties. Experience of health problems following hospital discharge was not a focus of this study.

The NICE (2006a) postnatal guideline recommends that after 24hrs of giving birth, women should be asked about their experience of common problems including perineal pain, urinary symptoms, bowel function, fatigue, headache and back pain with advice then given on their management and level of referral if any problems are reported. In addition to physical symptoms, psychological and psychiatric health problems such as onset of depression also have to be considered. Robertson et al (2004) completed a systematic review of risk factors for the development of depression and presented the outcomes in order of magnitude of effect size. These were depression or anxiety during pregnancy, life events such as bereavement, poor social support, previous history of depression, neuroticism and poor marital relationship. Low socio-economic status and obstetric factors had small effect sizes. The method used to assess depression in their review was not described, other than it had to have 'proven reliability'. The NICE 2007 mental health guideline found eight additional studies published since the Robertson et al (2004) review that largely supported the findings of the earlier studies.

Recent studies have examined whether there is a link between postnatal weight retention and psychological health. In one prospective cohort study from the US, 850 women completed the Edinburgh Postnatal Depression Scale (EPDS) at 20 weeks gestation and six months postnatal (Herring et al 2008). An EPDS score ≥12 indicated probable depression. Associations between antenatal and postnatal depression and substantial weight retention (at least 5 kg) were examined one year after the birth. The results found:

- 736 women (87%) were not depressed during or after pregnancy
- 55 women (6%) experienced antenatal depression only
- 22 women (3%) experienced both antenatal and postpartum depression
- 37 (4%) experienced postpartum depression only.

At one year, women retained a mean weight of 0.6 kg; 12% of women retained at least 5 kg. In multivariate logistic regression analysis, new onset postpartum depression was associated with more than a doubling of risk of retaining at least 5 kg (OR 2.54, 95% CI, 1.06, 6.09). Antenatal depression, either alone or in combination with postpartum depression, was not associated with substantial weight retention. A meta-analysis of studies which had examined associations between obesity and psychological morbidity in the general population found weak evidence of an association, with many of the 24 studies considered in the review methodologically poor (Atlantis and Baker 2008).

Current NICE (2006a) postnatal guidance includes:

"at each postnatal contact, women should be asked about their emotional well-being, what family and social support they have and their usual coping strategies for dealing with day-to-day matters".

The antenatal and postnatal mental health guideline (NICE 2007b) recommends that women are asked three questions at their first contact with primary care, at their booking visit, then 4 to 6 weeks, and finally at 3 to 4 months. The first two questions identify possible depression:

(i) During the past month, have you often been bothered by feeling down, depressed or hopeless?

(ii) During the past month, have you often been bothered by having little interest or pleasure in doing things?

A third question should be considered if the woman answers 'yes' to either of the above.

(iii) 'Is this something you feel you need or want help with?'

Services for women with mental health needs remain fragmented (Rowan and Bick 2008), nevertheless midwives need to be aware of signs and symptoms and implement timely and appropriate referral if this is indicated.

Care following caesarean section (CS)

The rising CS birth rate has important implications for the planning and provision of postnatal care, however there is limited evidence to support the content and duration of effective care following abdominal birth. Prophylaxis prior to, or at the time of birth, could minimise postnatal morbidity, for example use of compression stockings low molecular weight heparin (LMWH), early mobilisation and broad spectrum IV antibiotics and clinicians should ensure these are implemented in line with current guidance (NICE 2004).

Few studies have addressed care following CS birth specifically. With respect to obese women, Leddy et al (2008) recommend a number of measures to implement during and after surgery to limit morbidity. These include closing the subcutaneous layer, as seroma formation and postoperative wound disruption can be decreased in obese women if subcutaneous tissues are closed using layers of running sutures, and delaying the removal of skin sutures until at least seven days postbirth to allow tissue to heal completely. The evidence base to support these recommendations was not provided. More research into CS wound management is required but midwives should ensure that women are informed of signs and symptoms of SSI and wound dehiscence (separation of the wound edges) and advised to immediately contact their GP or midwife if concerned. At each contact, midwives should observe the wound for localised pain and erythema, local oedema, exudate, pus and offensive odour and ask the woman about her general health and wellbeing. For obese women, particular emphasis should be given to explaining the need for good hygiene, to keep the wound area clean and dry. Additionally, although not based on trial evidence, it would appear to be good practice when washing to raise skin folds which could occlude the wound when sitting or standing (Bick et al 2008).

In addition to ensuring wound healing is progressing, pain relief needs should be discussed at each contact. If the woman has been prescribed analgesia on hospital discharge which is effective, she should be encouraged to continue to take this. If this is inadequate or she has no analgesia, paracetamol can be taken as required up to 4g a day in divided doses, or used in combination tablets with codeine based on local prescribing policy (Bick et al 2008). If pain relief needs continue to be unmet, referral to the GP should be made.

Infant feeding

There is emerging evidence that among other health benefits breastfeeding confers on a woman and her baby (Bick et al 2008), it may also protect against childhood obesity (Arenz et al 2004; Fewtrell 2004; Karaolis-Danckert et al 2008) although further evidence is required to support this. In 2008, the Department of Health published Healthy Weight, Healthy Lives which recognised the importance of nutrition during the early years and the important contribution of breastfeeding. However despite the protective benefits of breastfeeding, a number of studies have highlighted that women who are overweight or obese are less likely to commence breastfeeding than women of normal weight (Amir and Donath 2007) and if they do commence breastfeeding, they are more likely to cease earlier than women with a normal BMI (Baker et al 2007).

Researchers have questioned whether in addition to social and mechanical factors, such as difficulty with latching the baby onto the breast which could account for early cessation, if physiological factors affect lactogenesis and prolactin levels (Hilsson et al 2004). In one small study, researchers examined prolactin levels among 40 women who had given birth to term babies to test the hypotheses that a reduced prolactin response to suckling and higher than normal progesterone concentration in the first week after delivery could be the means by which maternal BMI can compromise early lactation (Rasmussen and Kjolhede 2004). Serum prolactin and progesterone concentrations were measured by radioimmunoassay before, and 30 minutes after, the beginning of a suckling episode at 48 hours and seven days after the birth. Prolactin levels declined between 48 hours and seven days. Women who were overweight or obese before conception had a lower prolactin response to suckling than women who were normal weight, at 48 hours but not at seven days. After conducting multi-variate analysis and adjustment for confounding by time since the birth and duration of the breastfeeding episode, only being overweight/obese remained as a significant negative predictor of prolactin response at seven days.

Given these findings, and the knowledge that women who are obese are more likely to have had interventions during their labour and birth, it is imperative that health professionals have appropriate skills and competencies to support those who wish to breastfeed to successfully commence and continue to exclusively breast feed for as long as possible. Following discharge, it is important that women are informed of how to access local peer groups or lactation consultants.

Weight reduction post birth

Effective postnatal care could not only minimize health problems but could also provide opportunity to influence positive health behaviour with respect to a woman's weight. Excessive weight gain and persistent weight retention during the first postnatal year are strong predictors of being overweight a decade later (Rooney et al 2002). It is possible that weight loss and graded exercise programmes could impact on subsequent pregnancy outcomes, although evidence of this is required. One large Swedish study found that an increase in inter-pregnancy BMI was associated with a higher risk of adverse pregnancy outcome (Villamor and Cnattingius 2006). In addition to dietary advice, women should be advised to include regular physical exercise in their daily lives. Gentle exercise such as walking can be achieved by taking their baby out in the buggy, with small intervention studies showing such exercise can be safe and promote weight loss (Oken et al 2007).

Implications for health service resource use

Despite routine provision of postnatal services across the primary and secondary care sectors, there is limited information on resource use in terms of number of midwifery contacts, health staff costs or service utilisation including re-admission to hospital. MacArthur et al (2002, 2003) included a cost-effectiveness analysis as part of their RCT, which is an important consideration if the new model of care were to be adopted as standard practice. The comparative cost of delivering postnatal care between the trial groups was close, based on women's estimates of visit frequency. The extra intervention costs (for longer visits and the postnatal check by the intervention group midwives) were balanced by the slightly lower rates of GP home visits and fewer GP postnatal checks during the 12 months following the birth. Overall costs were equivalent indicating that the intervention model was cost effective as maternal outcomes were better. Petrou and Glazener (2002) looked at acute and secondary care health utilisation data for over 1200 women during the first two months postpartum, taking data from medical records, self complete questionnaires and hospital discharge records. There were significant differences in initial hospitalisation costs (based on 1999–2000 cost data) between the different modes of delivery groups (spontaneous vaginal delivery costing £1431, instrumental vaginal delivery £1970, CS birth £2924, P<0.001). There were also significant differences in the cost of hospital re-admissions, community midwifery care and GP care between the three groups. However, total post-discharge health care costs did not vary significantly by mode of delivery. Total health care costs were estimated at

£1698 for a spontaneous vaginal delivery, £2262 for an instrumental vaginal delivery and £3200 for CS (P<0.001). The study highlighted the economic consequences of alternative modes of birth which commissioners need to consider in terms of future service planning.

Additional pregnancy and birth costs are being incurred as a consequence of growing numbers of women who are obese when they become pregnant (Lashen et al 2004; Kerrigan and Kingdon 2008). In one US study, Chu and colleagues (2008) estimated the increase in the use of health services associated with obesity during pregnancy. Data from a large group practice health maintenance organisation were used to access data on over 13000 pregnancies between 1 January 2000 and 31 December 2004. Women were categorized as:

- Underweight (BMI <18.5)
- Normal (BMI 18.5 to 24.9)
- Overweight (BMI 25.0 to 29.9)
- Obese (BMI 30.0 to 34.9)
- Very obese (BMI 35.0 to 39.9)
- Extremely obese (BMI ≥40.0).

The primary outcome was mean length of hospital stay for delivery. After adjustment for age, ethnic group, level of education, and parity, the mean (±SE) length of hospital stay for delivery was significantly (P<0.05) greater among women who were overweight (3.7±0.1 days), obese (4.0±0.1 days), very obese (4.1±0.1 days), and extremely obese (4.4±0.1 days) than among women with normal BMI (3.6±0.1 days). Obesity was associated with significantly more antenatal fetal tests, ultrasound examinations, prescriptions for medication and antenatal visits. Obesity was also associated with significantly fewer antenatal visits with nurse practitioners. Most of the increase in length of stay associated with higher BMI was related to increased rates of CS births and obesity related high risk conditions.

Researchers from the North East of England interviewed 33 maternity and obstetric healthcare professionals with personal experience of managing the care of obese pregnant women from 16 local maternity units. Clinicians were asked for their views on the impact of maternal obesity on their services, the facilities required to care for them, and what existing services were available to care for obese women (Heslehurst et al 2007). Analysis identified five dominant themes relating to service delivery; booking appointments, equipment, care requirements, complications and restrictions, and current and future management of care. Other issues were associated with managing the care of obese women in pregnancy safely, including appropriate resources, need for multi-disciplinary care input to manage co-existing morbidities and restricted care options and choice for women who were obese.

The views of women

It is only recently that researchers have begun to realise the importance of obtaining the views of health service users, and evidence of the perspectives of women's experiences of postnatal care can be useful for informing revisions to care (Beake et al 2005). Few studies to date have asked women who are overweight or obese for their views of their maternity care, including aspects of care they found supportive or negative to meet their health or support needs. Nyman and colleagues (2007) in a small phenomenological study from Sweden interviewed 10 women with a BMI of ≥34 about their experiences of pregnancy and post birth care. Most reported negative experiences in their encounters with health professionals, with their weight forming the focus of their contacts and the perception that they were at risk of being discriminated. Clearly, if interventions to support obese women are to be effective and lead to positive health change, women's views are of paramount importance.

References

Amir LH, Donath S (2007) A systematic review of maternal obesity and breastfeeding intention, initiation and duration. *BMC Pregnancy and Childbirth* **7**:9

Arenz S, Ruckerl R, Koletzko B *et al* (2004) Breastfeeding and childhood obesity: a systematic review. *International Journal of Obesity* **28**: 1247-56.

Atlantis E, M Baker (2008) Obesity effects on depression: systematic review of epidemiological studies. *Int J Obes (Lond)* 32(6):881-91

Baker JL, Michaelsen KF, Sørensen IA *et al* (2007) High pre-pregnant body mass index is associated with early termination of full and any breastfeeding in Danish women. *Am J Clin Nutr* **86**:404-11.

Bhattacharya S, Campbell DM, Liston WA (2007) Effect of Body Mass Index on pregnancy outcomes in nulliparous women delivering singleton babies. *BMC Public Health* **7**:168 doi:10.1186/1471-2458-7-168.

Beake S, McCourt C, Bick D (2005) Women's views of hospital and community-based postnatal care: the good, the bad and the indifferent. *Evidence-Based Midwifery* **3**(2): 80-6.

Bick D, MacArthur C, Winter H (2008) *Postnatal care. Evidence and Guidelines for Management*. 2e Churchill Livingstone. London.

Central Midwives Board (1905) *Handbook Incorporating the Rules of the Central Midwives Board. 1st Edition*. Central Midwives Board, London

Chu S, Shin YK, Lau J *et al* (2007a) Maternal obesity and risk of stillbirth: a meta analysis. *Am J Obstet Gynaeol* **197**(3):223-8

Chu SY, Kim SY, Schmid CH *et al* (2007b) Maternal obesity and risk of cesarean delivery: a metaanalysis. *Obstet Rev* **8**:385-394.

Chu SY, Bachman DJ, Callaghan WM et al (2008) Association between Obesity during Pregnancy and Increased Use of Health Care *N Engl J Med* **358**:1444-53.

Confidential Enquiry on Maternal and Child Health, www.cemach.org.uk, accessed 18 March 2009

Confidential Enquiry into Maternal and Child Health. Perinatal Mortality 2005: England, Wales and Northern Ireland. CEMACH: London; 2007

de Boo HA, Harding JE (2006) The developmental origins of adult disease (Barker) hypothesis. *Aust N Z J Obstet Gynaecol* **46**:4-14.

Department of Health, Department for Children (2008) *Healthy weight, healthy lives: a cross-government strategy for England*. London, Department of Health; Department for Children, Schools and Families.

Ferrazzani S, De Carolis S, Pomini F *et al* (1994) The duration of hypertension in the puerperium of preeclamptic women: Relationship with renal impairment and week of delivery. *Am J Obstet Gynecol* **171**(2): 506-12.

Fewtrell MS (2004) The long-term benefits of having been breast-fed. *Current Paediatrics* **14**: 97-103.

Fretts RC (2005) Etiology and prevention of stillbirth. *Am J Obstet Gynecol* **193**:1923-35.

Gifford RW Jr, August PA, Cunningham G *et al* (2000) Report of the national high blood pressure education program working group on high blood pressure in pregnancy. *American Journal of Obstetrics and Gynecology* **183** Suppl:1-22.

Glazener C, Abdalla M, Stroud P *et al* (1995) Postnatal maternal morbidity: extent,causes, prevention and treatment. *Br J Obstet Gynaecol* **102**:282–7.

Goldenberg RL, Kirby R, Culhane JF (2004) Stillbirth: a review. *J Matern Fetal Neonatal Med* **16**:79-94.

Herring SJ, Rich-Edwards JW, Oken E *et al* (2008) Association of postpartum depression with weight retention 1 year after childbirth. *Obesity* **16**(6):1296-301

Heslehurst N, Lang R, Rankin J *et al* (2007) Obesity in pregnancy: a study of the impact of maternal obesity on NHS maternity services. *BJOG* **114**(3):334-42

Hilsson JA, Rasmussen KM, Kjolhede CL (2004) High prepregnant body mass index is associated with poor lactation outcomes among white, rural women independent of psychosocial and demographic correlates. *J Hum Lact* **20**:18–29

Horan TC, Gaynes RP, Martone WJ, Jarvis WR, Emori TG. CDC definitions of nosocomial surgical site infections, 1992: a modification of CDC definitions of surgical wound infections. Infect Control Hosp Epidemiol 1992; 13(10): 606-8. Johnson A, Young D, Reilly J (2006) Caesarean section surgical site infection surveillance. *Journal of Hospital Infection* **1**: 1-6

Karaolis-Danckert N, Buyken AE, Kulig M *et al* (2008). *H*ow pre- and postnatal risk factors modify the effect of rapid weight gain in infancy and early childhood on subsequent fat mass development: results from the Multicenter Allergy Study. *Am J Clin Nutr* **87**(5): 1356-64.

Kerrigan AM, Kingdon C (2009) Maternal obesity and pregnancy: a retrospective study. *Midwifery*, doi:10.1016/j.midw. 2008.12.005

Knight M, Kurinczuk JJ, Tuffnell D *et al* (2005) The UK obstetric surveillance system for rare disorders of pregnancy. **BJOG 112**:263-5.

Knight M, Kurinczuk JJ, Spark P *et al* (2009) Inequalities in maternal health: national cohort study of ethnic variation in severe maternal morbidities. *BMJ* **338**:b542 doi:10.1136/bmj.b542

Knight M, Kurinczuk JJ, Spark P *et al* on behalf of *UKOSS United Kingdom Obstetric Surveillance System (UKOSS) Annual Report 2007.* National Perinatal Epidemiology Unit, Oxford.

Knight M, Kurinczuk JJ, Spark P *et al* on behalf of UKOSS. *United Kingdom Obstetric Surveillance System (UKOSS) Annual Report 2008.* National Perinatal Epidemiology Unit, Oxford.

Ladner HE, Danielsen B, Gilbert WM (2005) Acute myocardial infarction in pregnancy and the puerperium: a population-based study. *Obstet Gynecol* **105** (3): 480-4.

Lashen H, Fear K, Sturdee DW (2004) Obesity is associated with increased risk of first trimester and recurrent miscarriage: matched case-control study. *Human Reproduction* **19**: 1644–6.

Leddy MA, Power ML, Schulkin J (2008) The Impact of Maternal Obesity on Maternal and Fetal Health. *Rev Obstet Gynecol* **1**(4):170-8.

Lewis G (2007) *Saving Mothers' Lives: Reviewing maternal deaths to make motherhood safer – 2003-2005.* The Seventh Report of the Confidential Enquiries into Maternal Deaths in the United Kingdom.

MacArthur C, Lewis M, Knox EG (1991) *Health After Childbirth.* The Stationery Office.

MacArthur C, Winter H, Bick D *et al (*2002) Effects of redesigned community postnatal care on women's health 4 months after birth: a cluster randomised controlled trial. *The Lancet*; **359**: 378-85.

MacArthur C, Winter HR, Bick DE. *et al* (2003) *Redesigning postnatal care; a randomised controlled trial of protocol based, midwifery led care focused on individual women's physical and psychological health needs.* NHS R and D, NCC HTA.

Mander R, Smith GD (2008) Saving Mothers' Lives (formerly Why Mothers die): reviewing maternal deaths to make motherhood safer 2003-2005. *Midwifery* **24**(1):8-12.

Marchant S, Garcia J (1995) *What are we doing in the postnatal check?* Br J Midwif **3**:34–8.

Mousa, HA, Alfirevic Z (2002) Major postpartum hemorrhage: survey of maternity units in the United Kingdom. *Acta Obstetricia et Gynecologica Scandinavica* **81** (8): 727-30.

National Institute for Health and Clinical Excellence (2006a) *Postnatal care: Routine postnatal care of women and their babies*. NICE clinical guideline 37.

National Institute for Health and Clinical Excellence (2006b) *Obesity. The prevention, identification, assessment and management of overweight and obesity in adults and children*. NICE clinical guideline 43.

National Institute for Health and Clinical Excellence (2007a) *Intrapartum care. Care of healthy women and their babies during childbirth*. NICE clinical guideline 55.

National Institute for Health and Clinical Excellence (2007b). *Antenatal and postnatal mental health: Clinical management and service guidance*. NICE clinical guideline 45.

National Institute for Health and Clinical Excellence (2008a) *Antenatal care. Routine care for the healthy pregnant woman. Second Edition*. NICE clinical guideline 62.

National Institute for Health and Clinical Excellence (2008b) *Diabetes in pregnancy: management of diabetes and its complications from pre-conception to the postnatal period*. NICE clinical guideline 63.

National Institute for Health and Clinical Excellence (2008c) *Surgical site infection. Prevention and treatment of surgical site infection*. NICE clinical guideline 74.

Nyman MK, Prebensen K, Flensner EM *et al* (2009) *Obese women's experiences of encounters with midwives and physicians during pregnancy and childbirth* doi:10.1016/j.midw.10.008

Pattinson RC, Buchmann E, Mantel GD *et al* (2003) Can enquiries into severe acute maternal morbidity act as a surrogate for maternal death enquiries? *BJOG* **110**:889-93.

Penney G, Kernaghan D, Brace V (2007) Severe maternal morbidity - the Scottish experience 2003 to 2005. Chapter 20 in: Lews G (Ed). *Saving Mothers' Lives: Reviewing maternal deaths to make motherhood safer – 2003-2005*. The Seventh Report of the Confidential Enquiries into Maternal Deaths in the United Kingdom.

Petrou S, Glazener c (2002) The economic costs of alternative modes of delivery during the first two months postpartum: results from a Scottish observational study. *BJOG* **109**(2):214-7.

Oken E, Taveras EM, Folasade AP (2007) Television, Walking, and Diet: Associations with Postpartum Weight Retention. *Am J Prev Med* **32**(4): 305–11.

Rajasingam D, Seed PT, Briley AL *et al* (2009) A prospective study of pregnancy outcome and biomarkers of oxidative stress in nulliparous obese women. *Am J Obstet Gynecol* **200**:395 e1-395.e9.

Rasmussen KM, Kjolhede CL (2004) Prepregnant Overweight and Obesity Diminish the Prolactin Response to Suckling in the First Week Postpartum. *Pediatrics* **113**: e465-71

Redshaw M, Rowe R, Hockley C, Brocklehurst P (2007). *Recorded delivery: national survey of women's experience of maternity care 2006*. National Perinatal Epidemiology Unit, University of Oxford.

Roberts CL, Ford B, Algert C *et al* (2009) Trends in adverse maternal outcomes during childbirth: a population-based study of severe maternal morbidity. *BMC Pregnancy and Childbirth* 9:7 doi:10.1186/1471-2393-9-7.

Robertson E, Grace S, Wallington T *et al* (2004) Antenatal risk factors for postpartum depression: a synthesis of recent literature. *Gen Hosp Psychiatry* 26: 289-95.

Rooney B, Schauberger C (2002) Excess pregnancy weight gain and long-term obesity: one decade later. *Obstet Gynecol* **100**:245-52.

Rowan C, Bick D (2008) *A* survey of perinatal mental health services in two English Strategic Health Authorities. *Evidence Based Midwifery.* **6** (4): 76–82.

Royal College of Obstetricians and Gynaecologists (2007) *Thromboembolic disease in pregnancy and the puerperium: Acute Management.* Green Top Guideline No.28.

Schrauwers C, Dekker G (2009). Maternal and perinatal outcome in obese pregnant patients *The Journal of Maternal-Fetal & Neonatal Medicine.* **22** (3): 218-26

Stothard KJ, Tennant PW, Bell R, Rankin J (2009) Maternal overweight and obesity and the risk of congenital anomalies: a systematic review and meta-analysis. *JAMA* **301** (6): 636-50.

The Information Centre (2009) *National Maternity Statistics England 2007–2008.*

Usha Kiran TS, Hemmadi S, Bethel J *et al* (2005) Outcome of pregnancy in a woman with an increased body mass index. *BJOG* **112**(6):768-72

Welsh Healthcare Associated Infections Programme (2006) *Caesarean Section Surgical Site Infection Surveillance. All Wales Annual Report 2006.* National Public Health Service for Wales.

Ward VP, Charlett A, Fagan J *et al* (2008) Enhanced surgical site infection surveillance following caesarean section: experience ofa multicentre collaborative post-discharge system. *Journal of Hospital Infection* **70**: 166–73

Waterstone M, Bewley S, Wolfe C. (2001) *I*ncidence and predictors of severe obstetric morbidity: case-control study. *BMJ* **322**:1089-94.

Waterstone M, Wolfe C, Hooper R *et al* (2003) Postnatal morbidity after childbirth and severe obstetric morbidity. *BJOG* **110**: 128-33

Welsh Healthcare Associated Infections Programme (2007) *Caesarean Section Surgical Site Infection Surveillance. All Wales Annual Report 2007.* National Public Health Service for Wales.

World Health Organization (2003) *Vaginal bleeding after childbirth. In Managing Complications in Pregnancy and Childbirth: a guide for midwives and doctors.* Geneva, World Health Organization.

Villamor E, Cnattingius S (2006) Interpregnancy weight change and risk of adverse pregnancy outcomes: a population-based study. *The Lancet* **368**:1164-70.

Chapter 11

Obesity Related Lactation Problems

Cecilia Jevitt

Introduction

Obesity causes metabolic perturbations that persist past pregnancy and birth into lactation. More than a decade of research shows that obese mothers are less likely to initiate lactation, have delayed Lactogenesis II, and are prone to early breastfeeding termination. These can cascade into further problems including increased maternal weight retention, future maternal type 2 diabetes and hypertension, and childhood overweight and obesity.

Rasmussen et al (2006) surveyed lactation consultants across the United States and found that only 29% of 80 respondents believed that obese women were less successful with breastfeeding than normal weight mothers. In a second survey of 31 lactation consultants, 23% asked for a definition of obesity. This demonstrates an ongoing need to understand the potential problems obesity imposes on breastfeeding so that women receive knowledgeable support. This chapter reviews the physiological benefits obese women can accrue from breastfeeding, the prevalence of lactation problems related to overweight (BMI 26-30), obesity (BMI>30), and current understandings of obesity related hormones and their effect on lactation. Finally, evidence-based techniques for midwives to reduce the impact of overweight, obesity, and excessive weight gain during the antenatal and intrapartum periods, as well as methods for supporting lactation in obese women will be described.

The benefits of breastfeeding for women with raised body mass index (BMI)

Emerging research indicates that breastfeeding protects mother and infant against a variety of future health problems.

The effect of lactation on maternal postnatal weight loss and future obesity

In the United States, 43% of women exceed antenatal weight gain recommendations developed by the Institute of Medicine (Institute of Medicine 2009; National Research Council 2007). Recommended antenatal weight gain includes approximately 2.27 kg stored fat meant to be energy reserves for lactation. Obese women enter pregnancy with sufficient fat stores for lactation yet are prone to excessive antenatal weight gain. This excess weight is difficult to lose and predisposes women to increased obesity.

Breastfeeding has higher energy requirements than pregnancy, utilising 400-500 kcal each day. Before the start of the obesity epidemic in post-industrialised nations, mothers lost body weight and subcutaneous fat during the postnatal period, with lactating mothers and undernourished mothers having higher weight losses. Higher daily energy expenditures through physical activity or work are associated with postnatal weight loss. Obese mothers who do not breastfeed, who breastfeed for short periods of time, and who have reduced stamina and mobility for physical activity, may not return to their pregravid weights during the first six months postnatal. This excess weight may persist longer than six months but most studies only follow women for six months postnatal. A Cochrane review (Adegboye and Lourenco 2009) of weight reduction after childbirth found that calorie reduction alone was effective in reducing excess weight. Calorie reduction combined with exercise was also effective for postnatal weight loss but exercise alone was not effective. This review did not include lactation as a weight loss variable.

Lactating women most often reduce physical activity thereby conserving energy and body weight (Winkvist and Rasmussen 1994). Weight accumulated with increasing age and parity confounds the effect of lactation on postnatal weight loss. These factors may partially explain the finding that the effect of lactation on postnatal weight loss is small for multiparous women in developing countries (Coitinho et al 2001). Primiparous women in this study lost an average of 300g for each month of predominant breastfeeding.

Baker et al (2008) completed more than 62 000 interviews of women selected from the Danish National Birth Cohort. Approximately half the interviews were done at six months postnatal and half at 18 months. The interviews examined breastfeeding and postnatal weight retention. Lactating primiparous women had greater weight losses than multiparous women, with breastfeeding being associated with lower weight retention in all BMI categories. The researchers created a model that suggested that for antenatal weight gains up to approximately 12 kg, exclusive breastfeeding for six months could eliminate postnatal weight retention.

A smaller study in the State of Georgia, US, had a similar conclusion (Hatsu 2008). Twenty-four participants were followed for 12 months postpartum; 17 exclusively breastfed for six months while seven used mixed feeding methods. The women who exclusively breastfed for six months lost more weight than the mixed feeding mothers, even though they consumed more daily calories.

Some women choose to increase physical exercise while lactating to augment weight loss. In one study (Lovelady et al 2000), lactating mothers were randomly assigned to a group that restricted intake by 500 calories a day and exercised 45 minutes four days a week or a control group, who neither restricted intake nor exercised more than once a week. After 10 weeks, the intervention group lost four times more weight and fat mass than the control group with no significant effect on infant growth. The effect of lactation on postnatal weight loss seems to end at about six months postnatal (Barbosa et al, 1997).

Calorie restriction to produce postnatal weight loss in lactating women is safe for the infant. Twenty-one average weight and 19 overweight Otomi Indians were studied for six months postnatal in Mexico (Barbosa, et al, 1997). All women lost weight over six months postnatal. Negative energy balance did not affect milk composition or nutrients, nor did it lower milk production or infant growth velocity. Two studies (Lovelady et al 2000; McCrory 2001) used randomised interventions to show that breastfed infants of overweight mothers, who dieted and exercised to lose an average of 0.5 kg/week, had normal growth. Moderate exercise compared to sitting did not change the immunologic properties of breast milk as measured by IgA, lactoferrin or lysozyme levels in a third study (Lovelady et al 2003).

The effect of lactation on future maternal metabolic syndrome

Pregnancy has been blamed for the accumulation of abdominal fat, weight retention contributing to obesity, and decreased high density lipoproteins. Improved analysis methods that take prepregnancy risk factors such as obesity into account and control for age and parity are expanding knowledge about the metabolic effects of pregnancy and lactation. Metabolic syndrome is defined as a clustering of insulin resistance, dyslipidemia, hypertension and obesity. A secondary analysis of the US Third National Health and Nutrition Examination Survey including 4699 women found that the more children women had, the higher the rates of metabolic syndrome were (Cohen et al 2006). A history of breastfeeding was associated with decreased metabolic syndrome. Higher BMIs decreased the strength of the association between breastfeeding suggesting that weight is a mediator of the effects of parity and lactation on metabolic syndrome risk.

Investigators used the ongoing multicenter US Coronary Artery Risk Development in Young Adults (CARDIA) Study to examine the effect of lactation on future metabolic risk factors (Gunderson 2007a). The three year prospective study excluded women with chronic diseases and multiple pregnancies. More than 1000 women were divided into three groups: women not pregnant during the three years; women who were pregnant during the three years but did not breastfeed; and women who were pregnant during the three years, breastfed for any duration and weaned the baby. As in previous studies, pregnancy was associated with weight retention and lower high density lipoprotein. However breastfeeding, especially breastfeeding for at least three months, was associated with increased low density lipoproteins, more favorable lipid profiles, postnatal weight loss and lower fasting plasma glucose.

A second multisite study (Ram et al 2008) compared 1620 midlife women, aged 42-52 years, who had previously breastfed with 896 who had not, and examined the prevalence of metabolic syndrome. The duration of lactation reduced the prevalence of metabolic syndrome in a dose-response manner. That is to say, the longer women had breastfed, the lower their risk for hypertension, abdominal obesity, impaired fasting glucose, and dyslipidemia.

The effect of lactation on future maternal type 2 diabetes

If abdominal obesity, dyslipidemia, and impaired fasting glucose are associated with type 2 diabetes and breastfeeding reduces risk for those conditions, does breastfeeding reduce the incidence of maternal type 2 diabetes? The evidence isn't clear. Lactation burns calories and diverts about 50 grams of glucose a day into milk synthesis using non-insulin mediated pathways in the mammary glands. Because of these metabolic changes, lactating women have lower blood glucose levels, lower insulin levels, yet higher rates of glucose production and lipolysis than non-lactating women. Few studies of women with prior gestational diabetes examine lactation (Gunderson 2007b). However, The US Nurses' Health Study found that increasing duration of breastfeeding reduced the risk of type 2 diabetes. For each year of lactation, the risk of gestational diabetes was reduced by 15% (Stuebe et al 2005).

The effect of lactation on future child obesity

The association between bottle feeding and childhood obesity is a compelling reason to help obese mothers overcome lactation difficulties. Silliman and Kretchmer (1995) found that obese women give birth to infants of higher adiposity (r=0.37, p <0.05); however by 6 weeks postnatal this relationship no longer existed in the 37 mother-infant dyads studied. Whitaker (2004) conducted a retrospective cohort study of 8494 low-income children who were enrolled in the Women's, Infant's, and Children's Supplemental Food Program and followed for 24 to 59 months. By 4 years of age, 24.1% of the children were obese (BMI >95th percentile for age and gender) if their mothers were obese in the first trimester of pregnancy. Neither Silliman nor Whitaker analysed the method of infant feeding in relationship to future weight. Breastfeeding for more than 4 months significantly reduced the future risk of obesity for infants of obese mothers in two studies. Baker et al (2004) used data from the US National Health and Nutrition Examination Survey III (NHANES III) and found that current maternal weight was the strongest predictor of children's weight regardless of duration of breastfeeding.

Owen et al (2005a) performed a meta-analysis of 61 studies reporting the relationship of infant feeding to the risk of later obesity. The 28 studies (298900 subjects) that could be compared using odds ratios supported breastfeeding's risk reduction effect for future obesity (odds ratio: 0.87; 95% confidence interval: 0.85-0.89). Owen et al (2005b) repeated the meta-analysis this time using 70 studies (60 published and 10 unpublished for a total of 414750 subjects). Their second conclusion was tempered, stating "Mean BMI is smaller among breastfed subjects. However, the difference is small and is likely to be strongly influenced by publication bias and confounding factors."

Breastfeeding research results are confounded by intervening variables such as supplemental infant feedings, maternal recall bias, inconsistent timing of infant measurements, and maternal antenatal health and weight. However, the United States Breastfeeding Committee (2005) advises exclusive breastfeeding for the first 6 postnatal months because it "may exert a small but positive influence in reducing the risk for obesity in childhood and later life".

The effect of lactation on future childhood type 2 diabetes

Research is ongoing; however, in one small study of 80 adolescents, fewer adolescents with type 2 diabetes had been breastfed than those without type

2 diabetes (Mayer-Davis, 2008). The crude odds ratio for breastfeeding and type 2 diabetes was 0.26 (95% CI, 0.15-0.46).

Initiation of lactation in overweight and obesity

One of the earliest studies revealing reduced breastfeeding initiation by obese women used the 1995 Australian National Health Survey. Donath and Amir (2000) compared 1 184 women with pregravid BMIs of 20-25 to 254 women with BMIs >30, finding that 89.2% (95% CI 87.4-91.0) of normal weight women initiated breastfeeding compared to 82.3% (95% CI 77.6-87.0) of obese women. Overweight women (n=490) had an 86.9% initiation rate (95% CI 84.0-89.9). The differences remained significant after adjustment for smoking, maternal age, and other sociodemographic factors. A 2007 systematic review of lactation initiation by Amir and Donath confirmed that obese women have lower rates of breastfeeding initiation.

Hilson, Rasmussen and Kjolhede (1997) reviewed the records of 1109 mother-infant dyads without potential lactation complications such as preterm birth, insulin dependent diabetes, and fetal malformations. Multiple logistic regressions were used to examine the relationship between maternal overweight and obesity and successful initiation of breastfeeding before hospital discharge. Adjustments were made for parity, length of gestation, mother's age and education, economic background, caesarean birth, gestational diabetes (GDM), maternal smoking and participation in the Special Supplemental Nutrition Program for Women, Infants, and Children (WIC). The obese women in this study had higher rates of GDM, infants with higher birth weights and longer gestational ages, and an increased number of caesarean births compared to women of normal weight. Overweight and obese women attempted breastfeeding at the same rate as women of normal weights (overweight: OR=1.196; obese OR=1.108), however significantly fewer overweight and obese women were breastfeeding at hospital discharge (overweight OR=2.54, P<0.05; obese: OR=3.56, P=0.0007). This cohort was 99% Caucasian, eliminating racial/ethnic variations in obesity as a confounding variable. In a similar study of 587 Hispanic women and 640 Black women, researchers found that obesity was associated with reduced initiation and duration of breastfeeding in Hispanic women but not in Black women (Kugyelka et al 2004).

Li et al (2003) analysed 124 151 mother-infant pairs who participated in the Pregnancy and Pediatric Nutrition Surveillance Systems. Mothers were categorised using pregravid BMIs and the American Institute of Medicine's (IOM) 1990 guidelines for antenatal weight gain. Only 46.7% of this total group had a normal pregravid weight and 42.5% gained more weight during pregnancy than advised by the IOM. Although 46% of the women initiated breastfeeding, obese women, regardless of antenatal weight gain, and women who gained excessive weight during pregnancy were significantly less likely to initiate breast feeding than women of normal prepregnancy weights who gained within IOM recommended weight ranges (P <0.01).

Duration of lactation in overweight and obesity

Along with reduced initiation, overweight and obese mothers stop breastfeeding earlier than women of normal weights. The 1995 Australian National Health Survey demonstrated that, "At any point in time, the odds that a mother who had a BMI >30 kg/m2 will cease breastfeeding were 1.36-fold greater than the odds that a mother with a BMI of <25 kg/m2 will cease breastfeeding" (Donath and Amir, 2000). The overweight and obese mothers studied by Hilson et al (1997) had significant drops in the rates of exclusive breastfeeding over the first 30 days postnatal. The relative risk of early termination of breastfeeding for overweight mothers was 1.42, P <0.04 and was 1.43 for obese women, P <0.02. Continuing work with this population, Hilson et al (2004) administered a psychosocial questionnaire to 114 lactating women, did daily phone follow-up for the first five days postnatal, and documented duration of breastfeeding at eight to 12 months postnatal. They found that obese mothers intended to breastfeed for three months fewer than did normal or overweight mothers.

Li's previously cited study found that obese mothers breastfed their infants about two weeks less than mothers of normal pregravid weights (average duration 14 weeks). Although this effect seems small, it was adjusted for other confounding variables including infant birth weight, young maternal age, low maternal education, poverty, unmarried status, and smoking. Antenatal weight gain, independent of pregravid BMI, affects lactation. The IOM issued antenatal weight gain guidelines in 1990 and reaffirmed them in 2007 (*Table 1*). Exceeding IOM (1990) antenatal weight gain recommendations in any BMI category reduces the odds of successfully initiating or sustaining lactation in all weight categories but most significantly for obese women (p <0.01) (Li et al 2003).

Research examining lactation, overweight and obesity in mammal models

Research with lactating mammals gives insight into overweight and obesity's effects on human lactation. Dairy science literature from the 1970s

Table 11.1 Institute of Medicine recommended antenatal weight gains (1990)

Weight category	BMI range	Recommended pregnancy weight gain lb (kg)
Underweight	<19.8	28-40 (12.5-18.0)
Normal	19.8-26.0	25-35 (11.5-16.0)
Overweight	26.1-29.9	15-25 (7.0-11.5)
Obese	>29.9	At least 15 (6.0)
From: Institute of Medicine (1990) and National Research Council (2007)		

describes delayed lactogenesis, milk fever, ketosis, and mastitis in overfat cows (MacCormack 1978). Overfeeding heifers before puberty reduces the volume of mammary gland epithelial cells and increases the number of adipocyte cells (Capuco et al 1995; Sejrsen et al 2000). Kamikawa et al (2009) fed nulliparous, non pregnant obese mice a high fat diet for 16 weeks then compared breast growth and breast tissue to those of lean control mice who were fed a normal diet. Obese mice had larger mammary glands because of increased fat pads; however their mammary ducts were less densely distributed and had less branching. Furthermore, the ducts were incompletely lined with myoepithelium and were surrounded by thick collagen layers. The researchers postulate that leptin stimulates leptin-receptor expressing fibroblasts in the periductal regions which produce and deposit collagen around the ducts inhibiting growth and branching.

Flint et al (2005) overfed rats to produce obesity in order to investigate obesity related abnormalities of lactation. Obese rats had reduced mammary duct side-branching and alveolar development during pregnancy. The amount of parenchymal tissue did not differ between lean and obese rats; however obese rats had increased amounts of mammary adipose tissue. Total DNA content in the glands of obese and lean rats was equivalent. Obese rats had reduced expression of α-lactalbumin, β-casein, whey acid protein on day one postnatal with β-casein and whey acid protein levels normalising over 10 days but α-lactalbumin remaining reduced. Based on these findings, Flint concluded that impaired lactogenesis is more related to impaired alveolar differentiation and development than reduced parenchymal mass. If humans have abnormal breast growth patterns similar to obese cows, mice and rats, childhood obesity may impair breast formation and development.

Diet also affects rat mammary glands. Rolls and Rowe (1982) compared obese rats fed high energy foods in addition to their regular chow, and normal weight rats fed only chow, finding that the suckling pups of obese rats had diminished growth and survival. Rats fed high fat cheese crackers in addition to their usual lab chow, which raised the percent of their dietary fat intake from 2 to 20% of the total weight of food eaten, decreased mammary gland lipogenesis by 50% (Munday and Williamson 1987). Milk produced by obese rats has higher fat concentrations but volume is substantially reduced (Rasmussen et al 2001a). Rats fed a high fat diet before and during lactation have difficulty initiating lactation and have low milk production associated with poor pup growth and high pup mortality rates (Rasmussen et al 2001a).

Rasmussen et al (2001a) attempted to reverse obesity related rat pup mortality by manipulating the fat content of postnatal diets. Lactating obese rats were divided into three groups: those receiving an unrestricted high fat diet, those receiving an unrestricted low fat diet, and those receiving a restricted low fat diet. The milk of the high fat diet rats was higher in lipids and lower in water concentration than the other groups. Milk production in the low fat diet group was 50% higher than in high fat diet group while the restricted, low fat diet group produced 12% less than the high fat group even though they mobilised stored fat for energy. The litters of the low fat dams with unrestricted intake had significantly higher growth than the litters of either the high fat or restricted, low fat diet rats. Rasmussen concluded that a low fat diet can mitigate the negative of effects of obesity and high fat feeding on lactation and pup growth.

Rasmussen et al (2001b) found that plasma insulin levels rise after 18 days of pregnancy and drop by three days of lactation in lean rats but not in obese rats. Plasma prolactin levels also rose from 18 days of pregnancy through three days of lactation in the lean but not the obese rats. Insulin and prolactin are essential for sufficient glucose availability during milk synthesis; therefore may be important hormonal variables in the failure of lactogenesis in obese mothers.

Delayed human lactogenesis

Human milk production is divided into two stages: Lactogenesis I and Lactogenesis II. Lactogenesis I encompasses the antenatal breast growth and development necessary for milk synthesis and culminates in colostrum production. Prolactin is necessary for the onset of Lactogenesis II, copious milk production, which begins approximately 48 hours after birth. Progesterone suppresses prolactin; therefore, Lactogenesis II cannot occur until the placenta, the main source of mammalian progesterone is expelled and progesterone levels fall.

Based on their work with lactating rats, Rasmussen and Kjolhede (2004) investigated obesity and human lactogenesis postulating that the precipitous fall in progesterone levels following delivery of the placenta triggers copious milk production as it does in other mammals; therefore, the progesterone stored in excess adipose tissue of obese mothers might prevent the rapid drop in progesterone from triggering lactogenesis II. Progesterone produced by retained placental fragments is known to prevent milk production.

Prolactin and cortisol are co-factors in milk production initiation (Neifert et al 1981) leading Rasmussen and Kjolhede (2004) to additionally postulate that obesity blunts prolactin and cortisol production further limiting lactogenesis II. To test their hypotheses, the researchers studied 40 mothers of term infants (23 normal weight and 17 overweight/obese women). They measured maternal serum prolactin, progesterone, insulin, glucose, estradiol, and leptin levels by radioimmunoassay at 48 hours and seven days postnatal before, and 30 minutes after, the beginning of suckling. Progesterone, insulin, glucose, and estradiol levels did not differ significantly between normal weight and obese women. Prolactin baseline levels decreased significantly from 48 hours to seven days postnatal in both the normal and overweight/obese groups. The prolactin response to suckling was significantly lower (p <.05) in the overweight/obese group than in the normal weight control group at 48 hours but not at seven days.

Leptin is an appetite suppressing hormone produced by adipose tissue and the placenta. It functions as a growth hormone in pregnancy with maternal levels dropping at birth. Obese women are hyperleptinemic and possibly leptin resistant. Leptin inhibits oxytocin-induced contractions of the myometrium in vitro (Moynihan et al 2006). Rasmussen and Kjolhede (2004) measured leptin during lactation finding that leptin levels at 48 hours and seven days were significantly higher in obese women. The milk ejection reflex is triggered by oxytocin. Could high leptin levels in obesity inhibit lactogenesis by diminishing milk ejection?

In Hilson's (2004) qualitative study of 114 lactating women increasing BMI was significantly associated with maternal perceptions of delayed onset of lactogenesis II (OR1.08; 95% CI=1.0,1.2; p <.04). One BMI unit is approximately 2.27 kg. For each one unit increase over a BMI of 20, there was a 0.5 hour delay in the onset of lactogenesis II. For women with BMIs >35 this would be a 7.5 hour delay. This delay is clinically important, as lactogenesis II may not occur before postnatal hospital or birth center discharge. Once discharged, if women do not perceive the breast fullness characteristic of lactogenesis II, they may lack confidence in their ability to produce milk and switch to formula. Even a five hour delay in lactogenesis II (BMI of 30) could affect energy and hydration levels in newborns, particularly macrosomic infants and those accustomed to a hyperglycemic intrauterine environment caused by maternal hyperglycemia.

A French study (Mok et al 2008) matched 111 obese mothers with 111 normal weight mothers for maternal country of origin, maternal age, maternal income and education, and parity. Infants were greater than 37 weeks gestation and birth weights were similar. Infants were exclusively breastfed. Infants of obese mothers lost significantly more weight during the postnatal hospitalisation than infants of normal weight mothers and gained less weight during the first postnatal month. This difference in growth disappeared by the third postnatal month. This suggests that obese women do produce less milk than women of normal weights.

Researchers prospectively followed 280 women, finding delayed onset of milk production (RR 2.01, 95% CI 1.45-3.64, p=.002) and suboptimal infant breastfeeding behavior (SIBB) on day seven postnatal (RR 2.58, 95% CI 1.07-5.22, p=.035) to be significantly associated with a maternal BMI >27 (Dewey et al 2003). Delayed onset of lactogenesis II was associated with stage II labor >1 hour (RR 2.26, 95% CI 1.24-3.57, p=.01) and caesarean delivery (RR 2.0, 95% CI 1.00-3.31, p .05). Suboptimal infant breastfeeding behaviour persisted in the infants of women with BMIs >27 with those infants being three times more likely to exhibit SIBB than infants of normal weight women.

Nissen et al (1996) determined that women who had emergency caesarean surgeries lacked a significant rise in prolactin levels at 20-30 minutes after the onset of breastfeeding and had fewer pulses of oxytocin on day two postnatal than women giving birth vaginally. Chen and colleagues (1998) found that primiparity, long labor, and stress to the mother and fetus during labor and delivery were factors for delayed lactogenesis. Obese women are at high risk for prolonged labor and caesarean birth (Hilson et al 1997; Dewey et al 2003). Caesarean birth coupled with obesity has been associated with delayed onset of lactation in several studies (Hilson et al 1997; Chen et al 1998; Chapman and Perez-Escamilla 1999).

Clinical implications: evidence based lactation support for obese mothers

Antenatal preparation

Obese women require planned support to initiate and sustain breastfeeding. A thorough psychosocial assessment should be conducted at the first antenatal visit. Many risk factors for obesity are psychosocial in origin (*Table 11.2*) and can be ameliorated with targeted social support. Chronic poverty, for example, is associated with obesity for multiple reasons. Ensuring that women receive government food support may reduce the association of poverty to obesity.

Table 11.2 Risk factors for obesity that further complicate lactation for women with raised BMIs

- Low wage, inflexible, hourly work
- Early school leaving
- Minority racial/ethnic status
- Food insecurity
- Decreased access to nutritionally dense foods
  - few full service or discount groceries in neighborhood
  - poor transportation to grocers
- Excessive antenatal weight gain
- Depression

Advice on the 2007 IOM antenatal weight gain targets (*Table 11.1*) to prevent excessive weight gain must begin at the first antenatal visit for maximum effectiveness (Hilson et al 1997; Li et al 2003) (*see Table 11.3*). Recommendations based on pregravid or first trimester BMI require accurate measurement of height and weight and calculation of BMI. Maternal recall of height tends to be inflated while maternal recall of weight tends to be underestimated. Twenty-four to 48 hour nutrition recall can be used to identify nutrition patterns. Advice should center on adequate caloric intake of nutritious foods with sufficient protein and iron while counseling the mother to avoid non-nutritious foods, such as soda and candy, and high fat foods. Mothers should never be advised to lose weight during pregnancy.

Nutritionists can be a valuable source of educational support. Many obese women qualify for nutrition services as obesity indicates excess calories not adequate nutrition. The weight gain of obese women and those gaining excessive weight can be followed more closely with antenatal visits at one to two week intervals. Preventing excessive weight gain reduces the likelihood of fetal macrosomia and caesarean birth. Both further complicate the success of lactation for obese mothers (Hilson et al 1997; Dewey et al 2003).

Intrapartum support

Because excessive stress during labor and surgical birth can alter the initiation of lactation and delay Lactogenesis II (Chen et al 1998; Dewey et al 2003), intrapartum techniques such as ambulation and frequent position changes should be used to allow the birth to be as physiologic as possible. Pain management techniques that reduce the amount of newborn sedating medication, such as hot packs and acupressure, can increase infant alertness and enhance early sucking strength and coordination. Epidural analgesia

Table 11.3 Midwifery management at first antenatal visit to reduce lactation problems related to obesity and excessive antenatal weight gain

- Assess psychosocial risk factors for obesity and lactation problems
- Measure height with a stadiometer
- Measure weight and calculate BMI
- Advise target weight gain at lower end of US Institute of Medicine recommendations
- Take history of weight gain, previous loss with regain, gestational diabetes, type 2 diabetes, hypertension or hypertensive disorders of pregnancy
- Determine if eating disorder, such as bulimia, is present and refer for psychological counseling as needed
- Perform 48 hour intake recall and assessment and nutrition review
- Recommend low fat intake with sufficient calories to avoid weight loss
- Refer for nutrition counseling if eligible
- Perform diabetes screen using 50 grams carbohydrate if no existing diabetes
- Schedule frequent antenatal visits, every 1-2 weeks, to assess weight gain and intake.

may relieve recalcitrant pain. No evidence has linked epidural medications with suboptimal breastfeeding (Chang and Heaman 2005). Caesarean birth should be avoided. Obese women are at increased risk for post-operative wound infection and deep vein thrombosis. The time involved in postnatal management of both these conditions takes maternal attention and time away from breastfeeding and recuperative rest.

Postnatal support

Postnatal support begins with the assessment of the risk factors that can complicate lactation (*Table 11.4*). Obesity further increases the risks posed by most of these factors. Knowing the associated risk factors can prepare nurses and midwives to be proactive in preventing these problems.

Table 11.4 Risk factors for lactation problems that further complicate breastfeeding for women with raised BMIs

Adolescence	Postnatal pain
Single parent	Caesarean birth
Primiparity	Post-operative incision infection
Poor social support	Postnatal hemorrhage
Excessive antenatal weight gain	Postnatal separation from newborn
Excessive stress in labor	Newborn macrosomia
Stage II Labor exceeding one hour	Intertrigo

Immediate postnatal feeding

Every effort should be made to keep mother and newborn together including post-caesarean recovery periods. Obese women may need special bariatric beds and chairs to sit or recline comfortably while breastfeeding, particularly those with BMIs exceeding 40. Beds and chairs must be wide enough so that bed rails and chair arms do not restrict the arm movement of obese women or newborn positioning. While privacy is always a consideration in facilitating breastfeeding, obese women may be self-conscious about their weight in addition to breast exposure. Obese women also have increased risk for caesarean births. Those initiating breastfeeding postoperatively will need pain management and positioning help that keeps the weight of the newborn off the abdomen.

Newborns should be put to the mother's breast as early as possible postnatal to encourage early and frequent suckling which triggers prolactin and oxytocin production, potentially negating obesity's blunting of the prolactin response (Rasmussen and Kjolhede 2004). Oxytocin released during nipple stimulation also reduces obese women's increased risk of postnatal hemorrhage by causing uterine contractions that constrict endometrial arteries. Obese mothers should breastfeed on demand, approximately 10-12 times in 24 hours, until the onset of lactogenesis II has been established.

Early feeding is critical to the prevention of hypoglycemia in macrosomic newborns. Encouraging mothers to place their infants skin to skin will assist with the stabilisation of respirations, heart rate, and thermoregulation and conserve energy (Bergmann et al 2004). These measures reduce the risk of hypoglycemia for the infant while maintaining close proximity to the breasts for frequent feeding.

Nipple/latch techniques

In addition to having larger breasts, obese women may have variations such as flat or inverted nipples which may further complicate the establishment of breastfeeding. Excess mammary adipose may stretch and enlarge the areola while flattening the nipple making it more difficult for the infant's mouth to encircle the areola and draw the nipple into its mouth. The mother with flat nipples can utilise a sandwich or C technique to insert her breast into the baby's mouth and elicit sucking. The mother makes a C of her thumb and index finger with the remaining three fingers in line with the index finger. The right hand is used with the right breast and left hand with left breast. The thumb is positioned on top of the breast and the index and remaining fingers provide support under the breast while drawing the breast away from the chest wall. The slight forward pressure generated by this movement may elongate the breast and push the nipple forward making grasp easier for the newborn. A mother with inverted nipples may benefit from pumping to evert the nipple. In time most women respond to pumping and infant sucking with increased nipple protractility. The use of a nipple shield to achieve latch, although controversial, may be an alternative and requires close follow up to assure adequate milk transfer.

An effective latch ensures that the mother receives adequate stimulation and the infant transfers milk effectively. The critical attributes of an effective latch have been identified as positioning, latch, sucking and milk transfer (Mulder 2006). To effectively breastfeed, the infant should be held facing the mother level with the breast, have a wide open mouth, flared lips, chin touching the breast and an "asymmetric latch" with more areola visible above the baby's mouth (Mulder 2006). Breastfeeding positions may need to be modified for maternal and infant comfort. The weight of large and heavy breasts should not rest on the infant's chest. Placing a towel roll under large breasts assists with stabilisation of the breast.

If engorgement of the areola is present then reverse pressure softening (RPS) can be used to soften the areola. This assists the infant in achieving an effective latch (Cotterman 2004). Reverse pressure softening has the potential to stimulate the milk ejection reflex and can be performed by a healthcare provider, the mother, or a significant other. Reverse pressure softening uses the pads of two fingertips to apply gentle inward pressure around the areola. It should be done prior to latching or pump use until the newborn masters latch.

If an infant latches but does not suckle, alternate massage can be used to assist with transfer of milk (Mulder 2006). Alternate massage is done by applying gentle downward pressure to the breast moving from the chest wall toward the nipple to assist with transfer of milk and breast emptying during pauses in infant suckling. This technique moves milk forward and can provide encouragement for the infant to maintain an effective suckling pattern while maximising milk transfer.

If the infant is not able to latch and feed effectively, then colostrum should be given to the infant in a manner that least compromises the transition to breastfeeding. Methods include spoon, cup or finger feeding. The infant should be held upright to feed with any of these methods and an amount of 0.5 ml can be easily swallowed by the infant (Walker 2006). Providing the infant an initial snack of colostrum may boost energy so that the infant achieves a latch and initiates sucking. Hand expression of colostrum may be more effective than pumping and allows for easier collection. Mothers should be taught and also practice hand expression before hospital discharge.

Milk Pumping

If mother and infant are separated due to illness, milk production should be stimulated by emptying the breasts every two to three hours using a hospital grade pump. Breasts replenish milk an hour after emptying, allowing for hourly pumping if needed. Some lactation consultants advise pumping breast milk one hour after the infant feeds to increase breast stimulation. The pumped milk can be fed to the newborn by cup after subsequent breast feeds. This technique might be useful for preventing delays in Lactogenesis II but has not been studied. Double pumping in addition to breast massage has been shown to produce better results for milk output (Jones et al 2001).

The standard 24mm breast pump shield may not sufficiently cover an obese breast, causing rubbing and strangulation with each pull leading to nipple damage. Ensuring that the breast shields provided are large enough will make pumping more effective and avoid nipple trauma. Most pump manufacturers make shields in three sizes and a nipple measurement tool to assist with shield fitting, equipment that should be available on all postnatal units. Information and support should be provided regarding breast pump use, storage and transport of breast milk, and infant feeding techniques. Mothers should be aware of community resources that provide rental or loans of breast pumps.

Post-discharge lactation support

Planning lactation support prior to hospital discharge, as well as providing close follow up, may be critical to continued breastfeeding (*Table 11.5*). Discharge lessons should consist of a review of infant feeding cues, duration and frequency of breast feedings, education regarding the identification of swallowing at the breast, indicators of adequate infant intake, and achievement of a comfortable and appropriate latch to assure effective transfer of milk. Parents should be alerted to upcoming infant growth spurts with increases in infant appetite that may make milk production seem insufficient for approximately 24 hours. Parents should also know that normal breastfed newborns, especially those who are macrosomic, may wake every two to three hours wanting to be fed. Giving parents a log, in which they can mark infant stools and urine along with breast feedings and daily breast assessments may assist with recognition of adequate output and early identification of problems. Once Lactogenesis II starts there will be an increase in the number of stools and at least 6-8 wet diapers a day. Contacts for breastfeeding assistance and local lactation consultants should be provided upon discharge.

In the absence of chronic disease such as heart disease or asthma,

Table 11.5 Intrapartum and postnatal midwifery management to reduce the effect of obesity on lactation

Intrapartum

- Use techniques such as ambulation, & frequent position changes to decrease labor stress
- Use nonpharmacological pain relief methods to increase newborn alertness and sucking strength
- Support physiologic birth to avoid surgical stress and postoperative complications

Immediate postnatal

- Limit maternal-newborn separation
- Support early and frequent suckling
- Facilitate newborn latch on
- Use bariatric beds and chairs when available
- Provide breast support with towel roll
- Teach mothers assessment of infant intake through adequate diaper wetting and stooling
- Teach and support mother in use of breast pump and infant feeding of pumped milk if mother-newborn separation is necessary

Following day 2 postnatal

- Encourage low fat intake of at least 1500 calories per day
- Teach signs and home management of intertrigo and infant thrush
- Encourage gradual resumption of physical activity to at least 30 minutes of walking daily
- Refer mother to lactation counselor or lactation support group if available
- Provide frequent community health visits, clinic visits or telephone follow-up to limit early termination of lactation
- Educate mother in availability of galactogogues and how to obtain

mothers may resume physical exercise gradually until they are walking at least 30 minutes per day which may be done in 10-15 minute increments. Physical activity helps burn excess intake if weight stabilisation or loss is desired postnatal. Obese residents of low income neighborhoods have been shown to walk more than residents of higher income housing areas (Stafford et al 2007). Safety may be a concern for women living in low income areas and must be taken into account when advising increased activity.

Overweight and obese mothers should also be encouraged to choose low fat foods during lactation (Rolls and Rowe 1982). Mothers may restrict intake no lower than 1500 calories a day to lose weight but should wait until lactation is well established (Baker et al 2004). Calorie restriction is more important to weight loss than the ratios of fat, protein, and carbohydrates (Sacks et al 2009). A Cochrane Review (Thomas et al 2007) however, found that low glycemic diets were superior in weight loss and lowering lipids. A low glycemic diet would provide a low fat diet. Pregnancy and a newborn's addition to the family are life events that change daily routines and personal values making them opportune times to introduce positive nutrition changes.

Galactogogues

Galactogogues, herbs or medications with evidence demonstrating their ability to increase milk production, should be the last resort when mothers feel that milk production is insufficient. Checking latch and sucking, checking nipple integrity, increasing feeding intervals, stimulating the breast between feeds with pumping, and increasing maternal rest should all be tried before galactogogue use. Given the potential delay in Lactogenesis II, midwives should be familiar with galactogogues.

Fenugreek is a traditional galactogogues herb used as a flavoring in Indian cooking. Fenugreek has anti-inflammatory properties and increases the activity of sweat glands. Milk glands are modified sweat glands and respond to Fenugreek. Fenugreek is widely available in capsules which are taken orally three times a day. The potency of the seed is variable but the effect should be evident in about 24 hours. Fenugreek gives a maple-syrup like odor to urine.

Metaclopramide is widely used in the US as a post-operative antiemetic and gastrointestinal tract stimulant. It is a dopamine antagonist which stimulates prolactin release from the anterior pituitary, as dopamine's prolactin-inhibiting effect is blocked. Metaclopramide 10 mg is taken orally two to four times a day, until milk production increases in three to four days, and then tapered off gradually over a week. It is secreted in breastmilk but considered safe. The dopamine inhibiting effect contributes to about 10% of women using metaclopramide feeling sleepy, fatigued or anxious. Women must be warned of these side effects and watched for incipient depression.

Domperidone is known as the Dom Perignon of galactogogues. It is another antidopaminergic related to metaclopramide that increases breastmilk production by increasing prolactin release. Domperidone has not been available commercially in the US since 2004 when the US Food and Drug Administration issued a warning about domperidone use and cardiac problems. Prior to that time, domperidone was used for decreasing emesis in infants, particularly those with failure to thrive. Domperidone can be obtained from compounding pharmacies in the US or ordered over the internet. Domperidone has no central nervous system effects for the mother because it does not pass the blood brain barrier. Little of it passes into breastmilk. The dose of domperidone is 10-20 mg orally three to four times a day with its effect being seen at day three or four.

Breastfeeding after bariatric surgery

Bariatric surgery with gastric banding or bypass is increasingly available to women whose BMIs exceed 35, who have been unsuccessful with other weight loss methods, or those with BMIs greater than 30 with co-morbidities. Clinicians can expect to care for more women with pregnancies following bariatric surgery as the substantial weight loss that occurs after bariatric surgery is essential in re-establishing ovulation and fertility in many obese women. There are case reports of B12 deficiency and failure to thrive in breastfed infants born after maternal gastric bypass surgery (Wardinksy et al 1995). Mothers lactating after bypass surgery lack gastric intrinsic factor to absorb B12. They will need multivitamin supplements with regular nutrition and infant growth surveillance and may need parenteral B12 supplementation (Wardinksy et al 1995).

The early postnatal period in women with prior breast reduction surgery

Obese women may choose breast reduction surgery to stop the shoulder and back pain associated with pendulous breasts. Those who have reconstructive surgery before childbearing and lactation will be unable to breastfeed as mammary ducts will be transected during the surgery. Women who have had breast reduction surgery should be watched closely in the immediate postnatal period as any milk glands remaining may initiate milk production and cause partial engorgement. Conservative measures such as ice packs, a tight fitting bra or breast binder, and ibuprophen for pain will decrease discomfort until the unemptied glands stop milk production, a period generally less than 72 hours.

Medications commonly associated with obesity during lactation

Table 11.6 lists classes of medication that are used frequently during breastfeeding for obesity-related conditions. Although total medication avoidance during lactation is an ideal, it is impractical. Poorly managed morbidities, such as infection or depression, will make breastfeeding burdensome and can lead to early weaning.

Table 11.6 Medications frequently used postnatally for treatment of obesity-related complications during lactation

Medication group	Obesity-related indication	Comments
Analgesic	Postnatal or post-caesarean pain	Ibuprophen compatible with lactation. Observe baby closely for sedation after narcotic use.
Antibiotics	Increased risk of caesarean birth and wound infection	Penicillins, ciprofloxacin, metronidazole & azithromycin considered safe during lactation. Avoid tetracycline. It stains newborn teeth.
Anticoagulants	Increased risk of thrombosis	Aspirin, heparin & warfarin are compatible with breastfeeding. Warfarin doesn't enter milk.
Antidepressants	Increased risk of depression	L3 options: Serotonin Selective Reuptake Inhibitors (fluoxitine, sertraline, citalopram). Paroxetine is safe for breastfeeding but is teratogenic in pregnancy.
Antihypertensives	Increased risk for chronic hypertension and preeclampsia	ACE inhibitors compatible with breastfeeding: enalapril, captopril
Anxiolytics	Increased risk for anxiety disorders	L3: buspirone
Hypnotics	Increased risk for sleep apnea and disturbed sleep	L2: zaleplon
Oral hypoglycemics	Increased risk of type 2 diabetes	L3: glyburide, metformin

L1= safest choice in drug class, L2=safer, L3=considered moderately safe

Sources: Buhimschi C & Weiner C (2009a and 2009b) & ACOG Practice Bulletin #92 (2008)

Intertrigo

Intertrigo, inflammation of skin folds caused by skin to skin or clothing friction, is a common problem of the obese breast. Intertrigo progresses from erythema and maceration to reddened plaques that may have fissures and exudates. Women may complain of intense itching, burning and pain as intertrigonous areas become secondarily infected with bacteria or fungi, most commonly candida. Although the obese breast needs a bra with firm support, care must be taken that the fit is non-constricting and that the fabric is light, non-synthetic, and porous. Following exercise causing perspiration, mothers must clean and thoroughly dry breast skin folds. Protective creams may be used as skin barriers (Janniger et al 2005). Using cornstarch as a drying agent should be avoided as moist starch may be a growth medium for fungi. Mothers should be taught the symptoms of candidal breast infections and infant oral thrush. Secondary infections often form pustules and should be treated with the appropriate antibiotic or antifungal agent.

Psychosocial needs of obese women during lactation

Obesity is associated with depression (de Wit 2009). Social criticism of excess weight as "unfit" may further erode self-confidence. Some evidence indicates that individuals who are chronically stressed eat to interrupt the hypothalamic-pituitary-adrenal stress-response system (Dallman 2003). Foods high in sugar and fat stimulate dopamine release yielding a sense of well-being; therefore, overeating may become a behavior learned to relieve stress. Additionally, stressful life events interrupt the discipline needed for weight management efforts.

When discussing dietary changes, midwives should affirm the nutritious foods that a woman eats while having the woman suggest one or two changes that she thinks she can make. A woman might, for example, replace drinking sodas with water. Replacement strategies may succeed better than advice to stop eating certain foods. Food preferences are primed in-utero and are culturally bound making them some of the most difficult behaviors to change. If eating certain foods gives women comfort, midwives must think about what behaviors can be used to provide comfort in place of eating. Oxytocin released during breastfeeding and endorphins released during physical activity both give a sense of well-being that might be useful in reducing comfort eating.

Given the increased rate of early weaning by obese mothers, first time breastfeeding mothers may require prolonged support and education about lactation and infant feeding, particularly if other family members are not experienced with breastfeeding. Mothers' perceptions that infants are not receiving sufficient breastmilk was consistently among mothers' top three reasons for early weaning. Skilled midwifery support can give mothers the knowledge and support they need to continue breastfeeding.

Conclusion

Midwives can reduce the risk of both maternal and childhood obesity by recognising maternal obesity and its potential effects on lactation. Lactation support begins at the first antenatal visit with weight assessment and nutrition counseling that optimises maternal weight gain and fetal growth. Physiologic labor support that reduces stress during labor and the incidence of surgical birth reduces obesity-related postnatal complications that might separate mother and newborn or suppress lactation stimulating hormones. Finally, midwives can provide on-going postnatal support that maximises breastfeeding success for mother and newborn and improves their health for a lifetime.

References

Adegboye A, Lourenco L (2009) Diet or exercise, or both, for weight reduction in women after childbirth. *Cochrane Database of Systematic Reviews* **3**: Article No: CD005627. DOI:10.1002/14651858.CD005627.pub2

American College of Obstetricians and Gynecologists (2008) Use of psychiatric medications during pregnancy and lactation, Practice Bulletin #92. *Obstet Gyne* **111**:1001-20

Amir L, Donath S (2007) A systematic review of maternal obesity and breastfeeding intention, initiation and duration. *BMC Pregnancy and Childbirth* **7**:9. http://www.biomedcentral.com/1471-2393/7/9 (accessed 5 May 2009)

Baker J, Gamborg M, Leitmann B, Lissner L, Sorensen T, Rasmussen K (2008) Breastfeeding reduces postpartum weight retention. *Am J Clin Nutr* **88**:1543-51

Baker J, Michaelsen K, Rasmussen K, Sorensen T (2004) Maternal prepregnant body mass index, duration of breastfeeding, and timing of complimentary food introduction are associated with infant weight gain. *Am J Clin Nutri* **80**:1579-88

Barbosa L, Butte NF, Villalpando S, Wong WW, Smith EO (1997) Maternal energy balance and lactation performance of Mesoamerindians as a function of body mass index. *Am J Clin Nutr* **66**:575-83

Bergmann NJ, Linley LL, Fawcus SR (2004) Randomized controlled trial of skin to skin contact from birth versus conventional incubator for physiological stabilization in 1200 to 2199 g newborns. *Acta Pediatric* **93**:779-785

Buhimschi C, Weiner C (2009a) Medications in pregnancy and lactation, part 1: teratology. *Obstet Gyne* **113**:166-92

Buhimschi C, Weiner C (2009b) Medications in pregnancy and lactation, part 2: drugs with minimal of unknown human teratogenic effect. *Obstet Gyne* **113**:417-42

Chang Z, Heaman M (2005) Epidural analgesia during labor and delivery: effects on the initiation and continuation of effective breastfeeding. *J Hum Lact* **21**:305-14

Chapman D, Perez-Escamilla R, (1999) Identification of risk factors for delayed onset of lactation. *J Am Diet Assoc* **99**:450-4

Chen D, Nommsen-Rivers L, Dewey K, Lonnerdal B (1998) Stress during labor and delivery and early lactation performance. *Am J Clin Nutr* **68**:335-44

Cohen A, Pieper CF, Brown AJ *et al* (2006) Number of children and risk of metabolic syndrome in women. *J Women's Health* **15**:763-73

Coitinho D, Sichieri R, Benecio M (2001) Obesity and weight change related to parity and breast-feeding among parous women in Brazil. *Public Health Nutrition* **4**:865-70

Cotterman K (2004) Reverse pressure softening: A simple toll to prepare areola for easier latching during engorgement. *J Human Lactation* **20**:227-37

Dallman M, Pecoraro N, Akana S *et al* (2003) Chronic stress and obesity: a new view of "comfort food." *PNAS* **100**: 11696-11701

Dewey KG, Heinig MH, Nommsen LA (1993) Maternal weight-loss patterns during prolonged lactation. *Am J Clin Nutr* **58**:162-6

de Wit L, van Straten A, van Herten M *et al* (2009) Depression and body mass index, a U-shaped relationship. *BMC Public Health* **9**:14. DOI: 10.1186/1471-2458-9-14. http://www.biomedcentral.com/1471-2458/9/14 (accessed 5 May 2009)

Donath SM, Amir LH (2000) Does maternal obesity adversely affect breastfeeding initiation and duration? *J Paediatr Child Health* **36**:482-6

Flint D, Travers M, Barber M *et al* (2005) Diet-induced obesity impairs mammary development and lactogenesis in murine mammary gland. A*m J Physiol Endocrinol Metab* **288**:E1179-87

Gunderson E, Lewis C, Wei G *et al* (2007a) Lactation and changes in maternal metabolic risk factors. *Obstet Gynecol* **109**:729-38.

Gunderson E (2007b) Breastfeeding after gestational diabetes. *Diabetes Care* **30**:S161-8

Hatsu I, McDougald D, Anderson A (2008) Effect of infant feeding on maternal body composition. *Intern Breastfeeding J* **3**:18. DOI:10.1186/1746-4358-3-18. http://www.internationalbreastfeedingjournal.com/content/3/1/18 (accessed 5 May 2009)

Hilson J, Rasmussen K, Kjolhede C (1997) Maternal obesity and breast-feeding success in a rural population of white women. *Am J Clin Nutr* **66**:1271-8

Hilson J, Rasmussen K, Kjolhede C (2004) High prepregnant body mass index is associated with poor lactation outcomes among white, rural women independent of psychological and demographic correlates. *J Hum Lact* **20**:18-29

Institute of Medicine Subcommittee on *Nutritional Status and Weight Gain During Pregnancy* (1990) Nutrition during pregnancy. Institute of Medicine. National Academy Press, Washington, DC

Janniger C, Schwartz R, Szepietowski J, Reich A (2005) Intertrigo and common secondary skin infections. *Am Fam Physician* **72**: 833-8, 840

Jones E, Dimmock PW, Spencer SA (2001) A randomized controlled trial to compare methods of milk expression after preterm delivery. *Archives Dis Child Fetal Neonatal Education* **85**:f91-5

Kamikawa A, Ichii O, Yamaji D, Imao T, Suzuki C, Okamatsu-Ogura Y, Terao A, Kon Y, Kimura K (2009) Diet-induced obesity disrupts ductal development in the mammary glands of nopregnant mice. *Developmental Dynamics* **238**:1092-9.

Li R, Jewell S, Grummer-Strawn L (2003) Maternal obesity and breast-feeding practices. *Am J Clin Nutr* **77**:931-6

Lovelady C, Garner K, Moreno K *et al* (2000) The effect of weight loss in overweight, lactating women on the growth of their infants. *NEJM* **342**: 449-53

Lovelady C, Hunter C, Geigerman C (2003) Effect of exercise on immunologic factors in breast milk. *Pediatrics* **111**:148-52

MacCormack J (1978) Fat-cow syndrome and its complications. *Vet Med Small Anim Clin* **73**:1057-60

Mayer-Davis E, Dabelea D, Lamichhane A, D'Agostino R, Liese A, Thoams J, McKeown R, Hamman R (2008) Breast-feeding and type 2 diabetes in the youth of three ethinic groups. *Diabetes Care* **31**:470-5

McCrory MA (2001) Does dieting during lactation put infant growth at risk? *Nutr Rev* **59**:18-21

Mok E, Multon C, Piguel L *et al* (2008) Decreased full breastfeeding, altered practices, perceptions, and infant weight change of prepregnant obese women: a need for extra Support. *Pediatrics* **121**:e1319-e1324

Moynihan A, Hehir M, Glavey S *et al* (2006) Inhibitory effect of leptin on human uterine contractility in vitro. *Am J Obstet Gynecol* **195**:504-9

Mulder PJ (2006) A concept analysis of effective breastfeeding. *JOGNN* **35**:332-39

Munday MR, Williamson DH (1987) Insulin activation of lipogenesis in isolated mammary acini from lactating rats fed on a high-fat diet. Evidence that acetyl-CoA carboxylase is a site of action. *Biochem J* **242**:905-11

National Research Council (2007) Committee on the Impact of Pregnancy Weight on Maternal and Child Health. *Influence of pregnancy weight on maternal and child health: workshop report*. http://www.nap.edu/catalogue/11817.html (accessed 2 September 2006)

Nissen E, Uvnas-Moberg K, Svensson K *et al* (1996) Different patterns of oxytocin, prolactin but not cortisol release during breastfeeding in women delivered by caesarean section or by the vaginal route. *Early Hum Dev* **45**:103-18

Owen C, Martin R, Whincup P (2005a) Effect of infant feeding on the risk of obesity across the life course: a quantitative review of published evidence. *Pediatrics* **115**:1367-77

Owen C, Martin R, Whincup P (2005b) The effect of breastfeeding on mean body mass index throughout life: a quantitative review of published and unpublished observational data. *Am J Clin Nutr* **82**:1298-307

Ram KT et al (2008). Duration of lactation is associated with lower prevalence of the metabolic syndrome in midlife—SWAN, the study of women's health across the nation. *Am J Obstet Gynecol*.**198**(3):268.e1-6.

Rasmussen KM, Wallace MH, Gournis E (2001a) A low-fat diet but not food restriction improves lactational performance in obese rats. *Adv Exp Med Biol* **501**:101-6

Rasmussen K, Hilson J, Kjolhede C (2001b) Obesity may impair lactogenesis II. *J Nut*r **131**:3009S-11S

Rasmussen K, Kjolhede C (2004) Prepregnant overweight and obesity diminish the prolactin response to suckling in the first week postpartum. *Pediatrics* **113**: 465-71

Rasmussen K, Lee V, Ledkovsky T (2006) A description of lactation counseling practices that are used with obese mothers. *J Hum Lact* **22**: 322-7

Rolls B, Rowe E (1982) Pregnancy and lactation in the obese rat: effects on maternal and pup weights. *Physiology & Behavior* **28**: 393-400

Sacks F, et al (2009) Comparison of weight-loss diets with different compositions of fat, protein, and carbohydrates. *NEJM* **360**:859-73.

Sejrsen K, Purup S, Vestergaard M, Foldager J (2000) High body weight gain and reduced bovine mammary growth: physiological basis and implications for milk yield potential. *Domest Anim Endocrinol* **19**: 93-104

Silliman K, Kretchmer N (1995)Maternal obesity and body composition of the neonate. *Biol Neonate* **68**:384-93

Stafford M, Cummins S, Ellaway A, Sacker A, Wiggins R, Macintyre S (2007) Pathways to obesity: indentifying local, modifiable determinants of physical activity and diet. *Soc Sci Med* **65**:1881-97

Stuebe AM, Rich-Edwards JW, Willett WC *et al* (2005) Duration of lactation and incidence of type 2 diabetes. *JAMA* **294**:2601-10

Thomas D, Elliot EJ, Baur L (2007) Low glycaemic index or low glycaemic load diets overweight and obesity. *Cochrane Database of Systematic Reviews* **Issue 3**. Art No.: CD005105. DOI:10.1002/14651858.CD005105.pub2.

United States Breastfeeding Committee (2005) *The importance of breastfeeding/human milk feeding in the prevention of obesity*. Raleigh, NC: United States Breastfeeding Committee.

Wardinsky T, Montes R, Friederich R et al (1995) Vitamin B12 deficiency associated with low breast milk vitamin B12 concentration In infant following maternal gastric bypass surgery. *Arch Pediatrics & Adol Med* **149**:1281-4

Whitaker R (2004) Predicting preschooler obesity at birth: the role of maternal obesity in early pregnancy. *Pediatrics* **114**:29-36

Winkvist A, Rasmussen K (1994) Impact of lactation on maternal body weight and body composition. *J Mammary Gland Biology and Neoplasia* **4**:309-18

Chapter 12

The Psychological Impact of being Overweight/ Obese during Pregnancy

Christine Furber and Linda McGowan

Introduction

As we have seen in previous chapters, the clinical management of overweight and obese women during the childbearing process has become a significant challenge for maternity caregivers in the 21st century. The epidemic of obesity that is so prevalent in the UK and many other developed countries seems to have emerged before research has been published that will help us to understand more clearly how to manage this.

Pregnancy is an important event in any women's life but for a woman who is already overweight or obese the changes that occur to her body may have significant consequences. Apart from the medical complications, how the pregnant woman views herself, her body image and self esteem, the perceptions she has about how others behave towards her, are factors that may impact on the quality of her pregnancy experience. It is important therefore that maternity caregivers have some understanding of the psychological issues and factors that may exacerbate negative feelings in order to plan optimum care.

In this chapter, an outline of some of the key aspects of the psychological factors that are known to be associated with being overweight and obese from the non pregnant population are presented. We have also summarised aspects of the research related to the psychological impact of pregnancy for normal weight, overweight, and obese women. Some of the key features related to the psychological impact of obesity during the childbearing process are highlighted from the authors' own research studies. A few interventions have been published that aim to support obese women during pregnancy and several of these incorporate psychological theory and principles in the design.

These have been summarised. Many of these interventions are focused on changing behaviour in order to promote a healthy lifestyle and aid weight control. The role of psychology theory to support behaviour change will be discussed. Finally, some recommendations for clinical practice that relate to psychological issues that may improve an overweight/obese woman's experience are suggested.

In this chapter, obesity is catergorised as body mass index (BMI) >30, overweight is BMI 26–29, normal weight is BMI 20–25, underweight is BMI <20.

We use the term 'maternity caregivers' to represent the differing health professionals involved in the care and management of obese women – midwives, doctors, health care assistants, for example.

The psychological impact of obesity

There appears to be limited published research relating specifically to the psychological impact of obesity during pregnancy. This is in contrast to a larger volume of research related to psychological impact of obesity in the non-pregnant population. It is worth reading a little about some of the studies with the non pregnant population, as the study findings will still have relevance for pregnant women.

The psychological impact of obesity in non-pregnant adults

Two main concepts have emerged from the literature that relate to the psychological impact of obesity in the non pregnant population:
1. Stigma
2. Psychological distress

Stigma

Puhl and Brownell (2001) summarised the literature and highlighted that prejudice and discrimination in education, the workplace, and healthcare settings were common experiences for those who are obese. Research with obese adults has shown that stigma in the form of negative verbal comments from family and friends (Friedman et al 2005; Puhl et al 2008), humiliating comments from health professionals (Merrill & Grassley 2008; Thomas et al 2008), and negative experiences in society in general such as total strangers staring and commenting on weight (Friedman et al 2005; Merrill andd Grassley 2008) and restricted access to social amenities because of size (Thomas et al, 2008), is widespread. A further review of the literature by Puhl and Brownell (2003) highlights that stereotypical beliefs about obese individuals, such as views that they are lazy, unclean and lack willpower, are not uncommon.

Psychological distress

The evidence suggests that those who are obese may be more prone to developing psychological distress such as depression and anxiety. Several cross sectional studies from the USA conclude that obesity is a risk factor for depression. Roberts et al (2003) followed up 2730 participants aged between 50–80 years over a 5 year period from 1994 -1999. Mental health was assessed using a validated tool that assessed Diagnostic and Statistical Manual of Mental Disorders, Fourth Edition (DSM – IV) symptom criteria for major depressive episodes. They found that participants who were obese when they entered the study were up to two times more likely to be depressed at five year follow up. This was one of the first studies to find an association between being obese and developing depression. Onyike et al's (2003) study with 8410 participants who completed the Diagnostic Interview Schedule which assessed depression and bipolar disorders indicated that obesity is associated with depression, especially if obesity is morbid (BMI >40) in females compared with males ($p < 0.00001$). Simon et al (2006) explored the mental health of over 9000 adults in 48 contiguous states of the USA using the World Health Organization Composite International Diagnostic Interview. These results indicate that there is an association between being obese and a range of mood and anxiety disorders ($P < 0.05$).

An interesting study by Hill & Williams (1998) explored the psychological well-being of 179 obese women by recruiting via a UK subscription magazine for women sized 16+ (UK clothing size). A questionnaire exploring body shape assessment, body shape satisfaction, dietary restraint, mental health inventory and self esteem was printed in the magazine. The effect of obesity with multiple measures was evaluated using analysis of variance. The results suggest that those with the highest BMI (>40) did not have the worst mental health, but they reported the greatest dissatisfaction with body weight, shape and appearance. This group also had the lowest self esteem, perceived they had fewer friends, and felt the least attractive. It is important to acknowledge the limitations of this study; the sample was mostly higher social class women who were able to subscribe to the magazine and the questionnaires were self-completed. However, obese women were specifically targeted and able to respond anonymously to potentially embarrassing questions.

The mental health of obese adults on weight loss programmes has also been explored. Friedman et al (2005) assessed the relationship between weight stigmatisation, beliefs about weight, and psychological functioning. They used the Beck Depression Inventory (BDI), Rosenberg Self-Esteem Scale (RSE) to explore depressive symptoms and self-esteem, and Stigmatising Situations Inventory to assess weight-based stigma in obese individuals at a residential weight loss house. The analysis reported that those with higher depression scores had more frequent weight stigmatising experiences. These experiences were found to be predictive of psychological distress and these included depression, general psychiatric function, self esteem and body image. Werrij et al (2006) assessed the mental health of overweight/obese adults seeking dietary treatment for their weight utilising the BDI, the RSE and the Eating Disorder Examination Questionnaire. Two groups were formed from scores using the BDI: one of 'non–depressed' overweight/ obese adults, and overweight/obese adults suffering from 'mild–moderate' psychological distress (the depressed group). A comparison of both groups indicated that the depressed participants were more likely to have lower self-esteem and be concerned about their shape, weight and eating habits than those not depressed ($p < 0.05$). These studies illustrate the importance of assessing depression when planning weight-management interventions as this could be a factor that influences success.

It is clear from the literature that being obese in today's modern society has far reaching implications for success in life, being accepted by family, friends and others, and mental well-being. It is likely that many overweight /obese pregnant women will be aware of some of these challenges before they encounter the maternity services. Negative past experiences may affect how they react and subsequently respond to maternity caregivers. Women with higher BMI, especially over 40, may particularly be more at risk of psychological distress.

Body image and pregnancy

It is worth considering the psychological impact of changes to the body that naturally occur in all women during pregnancy before we review the literature specifically related to obese pregnant women.

Body image, and changes to the body during pregnancy in normal weight women, has been extensively researched, especially by psychologists. Some studies indicate that pregnant women become progressively more negative about their changing body as pregnancy ensues. Strang and Sullivan (1985), for example, explored women's perceptions of their body retrospectively after the birth. In Canada, 109 women completed the Attitude to Body Image Scale at two weeks and six weeks after the birth. The results indicate that participants were happier with their postpartum body image than that during pregnancy (p <0.04). Other research indicates that women are happier with their body during pregnancy, than afterwards. A study in London, England, compared 50 pregnant women and 50 non pregnant women, and their weight concern in relation to eating behaviour and body dissatisfaction (Clark & Ogden 1999). The analysis suggested that pregnant woman felt that they had less dietary restraint, could legitimately eat more during their pregnancy, and were not as dissatisfied with their body shape when compared with non pregnant women.

More recent studies highlight the complexity of body image and pregnancy. A team in Melbourne, Australia, assessed body dissatisfaction and changes in body image over the course of pregnancy (Skouteris et al 2005). Eighty nine healthy pregnant women completed a range of questionnaires including the Body Attitude Questionnaire (BAQ), Perceived Socio-Cultural Pressure Scale and Public Self-Consciousness Scale, at three different times during the pregnancy period. Statistical analysis of the results indicated that pregnant women 'become accustomed' to the changes that occur in their body as the pregnancy progresses. Furthermore, the Skouteris et al (2005) study highlights some of the psychosocial risk factors that may affect body dissatisfaction in pregnancy including the presence of depressive symptoms, peer group pressure, and cultural expectations to be slim. More recently, the Melbourne researchers explored the relationship between depression and body dissatisfaction across pregnancy and the first year after birth (Clark et al 2009). The BAQ and BDI were completed at five points across pregnancy and up to one year after the birth by 116 women. The association between BDI the BAQ scores indicate that pregnant women have the least body dissatisfaction in the third trimester and this was associated with more depressive symptoms in this stage of pregnancy. When the analysis controlled for a range of factors, it was found that depression in later pregnancy predicted body dissatisfaction at six weeks postpartum (Clark et al 2009).

Johnson et al (2004) explored feelings about body, weight and eating behaviours compared to the past, and expectations for the future, with six pregnant women in the UK. This small but in-depth qualitative study also found that thoughts on body image vary throughout pregnancy. In particular, pregnancy was seen as a legitimate reason for gaining weight, and eating more, but as long as the weight gain was acceptable. Johnson et al (2004) highlight other factors about body image that are relevant when women are pregnant; that women are valued by society for their looks and ability to reproduce, for example. The changing body during pregnancy reflects these ideals, but the women in Johnson et al's study struggled to maintain the expectations of society and their role as a pregnant woman, with their personal experience of pregnancy.

Inevitably, changes to the pregnant body are visible to others. It is feasible that weight gain in pregnancy may contribute to feelings of stigma that has been highlighted in the non pregnant population. These studies emphasise that perceptions of body image and weight gain in pregnancy cannot be taken out of context of the society that women live in. For example, obesity is often not portrayed in a positive light by the media. To illustrate this point, Greenberg et al (2003) reviewed five episodes each of the 10 top rated fictional TV programmes on US TV networks during 1999-2000. Content analysis was used to analyse observations. Of 1018 characters viewed, only 14% of females were obese which is significantly less than in the general population of the USA. Furthermore, overweight and obese women were more likely to be seen as objects of humour (p <0.001), less likely to show physical attraction (p <0.05), have romantic interactions (p <0.05), and be seen as attractive (p <0.001).

The psychological impact of obesity in pregnancy

Of the published literature, two strands of research regarding weight and pregnancy have emerged, that of actual weight gain during pregnancy, and the experience of being an obese woman and pregnant.

Attitudes towards weight gain during pregnancy

Attitudes to weight gain during pregnancy have been shown to vary depending on a woman's prepregnancy size. In general, research has shown that the thinner the woman prepregnancy, the more positive her attitude will be towards the natural weight gain during pregnancy (Stevens-Simon et al 1993; Copper et al 1995). However, not all pregnant women are happy about ensuing weight gain in pregnancy.

In a small qualitative study carried out in England, Warriner (2000) interviewed 10 pregnant women to explore their views on being weighed during pregnancy. Warriner found that women who were strict about their weight before pregnancy exhibited distress when weighed in pregnancy. DiPietro et al (2003) conducted an observational study with 130 normal weight low risk women (BMI mean = 24.9) around 36 weeks of pregnancy in the USA. Almost half of the participants gained weight in excess of recommended guidelines for weight gain in pregnancy, whilst 40% gained within the guidelines. This study indicates that increasing pregnancy size has varying effects on women's behaviour. Around one fifth of the participants admitted to weight restricting behaviours such as not eating before an antenatal appointment, trying to hide the pregnancy early on, and deliberately varying weight gain each month. Furthermore, almost all of those who gained weight within the recommended guidelines were concerned about 'getting fat' at the end of the pregnancy ($p < 0.01$), and several felt unattractive due to their size ($p < 0.05$). DiPietro et al's study also explored positive feelings related to pregnancy. Thoughts associated with pregnancy being a heartening experience were associated with positive attitudes towards body image, greater weight gain, and participating in less weight-restricting behaviours.

It seems that increasing weight gain during pregnancy may be a matter of concern for some women. It is important to remember that some are prepared to go to significant lengths such as moderating their nutritional intake to limit this. This has implications for clinical practice and assessment of dietary habits and subsequent advice and information provided.

Being obese and pregnant – what do women say?

To date, only a few research studies have been carried out that explore the personal experiences and feelings of obese pregnant women. The majority of the published literature about obesity and childbearing has focused on the risks, outcomes, and management of pregnancy and labour. Of the few studies published that focus on psychological issues, it is apparent that being pregnant may have some positive feelings about weight for women who are larger than normal. However, many overweight/obese women describe childbearing as being a negative time in their lives. In this section, the published literature has been organised into three themes:

(i) The positive impact of being pregnant for overweight/obese women.
(ii) The impact on quality of life when pregnant and overweight/obese.
(iii) The effects of interactions with health professionals when pregnant and overweight/obese.

In the final section, some of the findings of a study (as yet unpublished) that the authors have recently completed are presented.

The positive impact of being pregnant for overweight/ obese women

The impact of pregnancy on overweight women's body image was explored by Wiles (1994; 1998). Wiles conducted two in-depth interviews with 39 women in late pregnancy and six weeks after birth in the late 1980s and early 1990s in England. Wiles found that several women were dissatisfied with their weight prepregnancy, whilst during pregnancy buying larger clothes and engaging in sports activities became increasingly difficult, for example. However, for some women being pregnant actually reduced negative feelings about their weight, by giving a feeling of liberation from the everyday perceived restrictions of their lives prepregnancy. Fox & Yamaguchi (1997) explored the relationship between prepregnancy body weight and body image in 76 normal weight/overweight primigravidae in the third trimester of pregnancy. A self-administered free response questionnaire and a modified version of the Body Shape Questionnaire was used for data collection in an antenatal clinic in London, England. Results indicated that overweight women were more likely to experience a positive change to their body image than the normal weight women (p <0.005). Responses to the free response questions indicated that overweight women felt less self conscious with their body image, and a release from the stigma of being overweight and pressure to lose weight. Confidence improved as overweight women felt more physically attractive. Some normal weight women also highlighted the release from the 'pressure to be slim' (Fox and Yamaguchi 1997). These studies indicate that pregnancy can be seen as a valid period in a woman's lifespan where gaining weight, and being overweight/obese is socially acceptable. Pregnancy may also have a positive impact on overweight/obese women's perceptions of their body image.

The impact on quality of life when pregnant and overweight/obese

Pregnant women's overall quality of life may be adversely affected by obesity. LaCoursiere et al (2006) explored BMI and depressive symptoms during pregnancy with postnatal women between two and six months after birth. This study was completed as part of the nationwide Pregnancy Risk Assessment Monitoring System across the USA with 3439 postpartum women randomly selected from the state of Utah. Data were collected by survey and analysed statistically. Although BMI was self-reported by the women, after controlling for marital status and income, they found that prepregnancy obesity was associated with moderate or even greater depressive symptoms postpartum (30.8% of obese women compared to 22.8% normal weight women). Furthermore, underweight and obese women reported emotional and traumatic distress during pregnancy and more depressive symptoms two to four months postpartum. This survey indicated that there is potential relationship between prepregnancy BMI and self reported symptoms of depression in the postpartum period.

A study of 220 Mexican women showed that obesity in pregnancy had a deleterious effect on the women's quality of life (Amador et al 2008). Using a specific quality of life scale (Short Form-12) they found that obese pregnant women had worse scores relating to the mental health components of the measure, than non-obese women, both at the beginning of pregnancy and in the last trimester. Furthermore, regression analysis showed that baseline BMI, weight gain, and complications in pregnancy (e.g. preterm birth, hypertension) predicted lower scores on the physical health component of this scale.

Although the research does not confirm that depression is caused by obesity during childbearing, caregivers need to be aware of these associations for their clinical practice.

The effects of interactions with health professionals when pregnant and overweight/obese

Unfortunately, as in the non pregnant obese population, obese pregnant women have described practices from maternity caregivers that have affected their confidence, and had a negative impact on their subsequent feelings and psychological state during pregnancy. For example, the authors conducted an exploratory study of mild–moderate psychological distress in 24 pregnant women in one maternity hospital in the north west of England (Furber et al 2007). Participants were asked questions to explore the source of their distress, and factors that exacerbated this, in semi structured interviews. One obese woman recalled her experience with an ultrasonographer during an ultrasound scan to assess fetal normality. She perceived that this interaction had left her feeling so humiliated to the extent that she did not want to return to the hospital again for antenatal care. See this extract from her interview:

> *"I got to the point where I thought I'm not going back. It was the scan appointment. The lady that did the scan had a student with her; she didn't even acknowledge that I'd walked into the room. All this was before I spoke to her. She scanned me. I asked her if it was alright and all she said was 'it looks like it. Wait in the waiting room I'll see you in a minute'. …. and she's discussing with the student, the fact that they couldn't scan properly cos of my weight and everyone in this waiting room …"* (Participant 17, 18 weeks pregnant) (Source: Furber et al 2007).

In Sweden, Nyman et al (2008) carried out an indepth qualitative study using phenomenological principles to describe obese pregnant women's experiences of their interaction with midwives and doctors during childbearing. Ten women with a BMI between 34 and 50 took part in interviews where they were encouraged to describe their experiences as openly as possible. The findings indicate that these obese pregnant women felt that they were living with a constant awareness of the size of their body. They felt that they were under close surveillance from caregivers during their pregnancy which made them feel uncomfortable and evoked negative emotions. These women found medical examinations frustrating as they were worried that the gowns that they were expected to wear, and equipment used, may not be big enough for them. Revealing their weight to caregivers, and their partners, was particularly embarrassing and shaming for these women. These women also described feeling guilty over putting their life, and that of their unborn child, in danger because of their obesity. They were aware that their weight put them at greater risk of thrombo-embolism and caesarean section, for example.

Furthermore, these women were very worried about the amount of weight gained during the pregnancy, and difficulties they may encounter after birth in losing this. In particular, they described feelings of fear of health professionals, especially midwives. Caregivers were described as treating these women less favourably than normal weight pregnant women. Anger and guilt was described at comments made suggesting that they should avoid pregnancy. These women described feeling hurt and sad when caregivers had difficulty examining their developing pregnancy because of their size. A lack of trust in caregivers was also described as the women perceived that their experiences of feeling contractions and baby movements were not believed. Women also described being reticent at challenging caregivers due to fear of receiving further poor care. Unfortunately, when the care received was perceived to be humiliating and offensive, the feelings of shame and guilt initiated further eating. Only when caregivers listened to the women, expressed consideration, and were helpful, did obese pregnant women in Nyman et al's (2008) study describe feeling relaxed and proud of their pregnancy.

The psychosocial impact of obesity on pregnancy

A recent qualitative study explored the psychosocial experiences of obese pregnant women in the third trimester of birth, and in the postnatal period around four to six weeks after the birth (Furber & McGowan, unpublished observations 2009). Nineteen women participated from one hospital in the North West of England. Semi structured interviews were carried out and questions explored feelings about weight, experiences of being obese and pregnant, reactions from caregivers and family and friends, and worries about weight to explore the psychological impact of being obese during the childbearing process. The data were analysed using framework analysis principles (Ritchie and Spencer 1994). The findings have provided further insight into the psychological impact of childbearing when obese. Several themes emerged during data analysis that indicates that being obese and pregnant has significant repercussions for psychological state.

Perceptions of body image were relevant. For example, most women interviewed 'normalised' their weight in comparison to others in society. These women were aware that they were larger than normal women but, on the whole, they were comfortable with their size. Being larger was not a significant hindrance in their daily life as, for example, buying clothes was not difficult. However, when they were weighed during the booking visit for assessment of their BMI, many women were shocked at their weight:

"It was a bit of a surprise to me to find out what my BMI was. I knew I'd put on weight, but when I see myself, I don't see an overly massive person" (Participant 4, interviewed at 34 weeks pregnant).

Anxiety was a feeling frequently described by these women. Although most women interviewed had little knowledge about the risks associated with obesity and the pregnancy, some women were anxious that their weight may have implications for the future. Some were concerned about developing gestational diabetes:

"I weighed more this time than I weighed when I got pregnant with my son by about a stone and a half. I was concerned cos I had gestational diabetes last time. I knew I really should have lost weight before I got pregnant" (Participant 9, interviewed at 30 weeks of pregnancy).

Others were worried about being able to care for their child in the future:

"Sometimes I think Oh God I need to lose weight. I've got a daughter, I've got to look after her and it might start affecting the way I look after her. I do get worried sometimes" (Participant 12, interviewed at 29 weeks pregnant).

Many of the women interviewed in this study described feelings of isolation. Isolation stemmed from the reactions of caregivers that provided care and support, but also from interactions with family and friends and experiences in the wider community. Although several women described encounters with their care givers that illustrated midwives and doctors were sensitive about their weight, some women described scenarios where they had felt humiliated and embarrassed from comments made, and care received similar to Nyman et al's (2008) findings. Similar to the non obese population, several women in the author's study described situations where they had felt victimised and blamed about their weight from family and friends, and the wider society. For example, one woman was interviewed shortly after the screening of a nationwide television programme about the trend in increasing size of babies at birth, and larger mothers. Immediately after the screening, this participant noted that others (neighbours for example) frequently commented on her size and likened her to the women in the programme.

What has been done to support obese pregnant women?

In the UK, the maternity services (funded by the National Health Service [NHS]) provide the majority of support for obese pregnant women. The assessment of pregnant obese women centres on medical parameters such as risk for developing gestational diabetes, hypertension and complications during the birth. At the booking interview, midwives assess BMI and are expected to provide advice on appropriate diet and exercise for optimum health in pregnancy (National Institute for Health and Clinical Excellence [NICE] 2008). The psychological assessment of pregnant women using validated screening instruments is contraindicated during routine antenatal care in England (NICE 2008). However, it has recently been recommended that midwives should explore pregnant women's mental health status using the Whooley questions (NICE 2007). Women who require further support for mental health issues should be referred to the appropriate service. Weight management during antenatal care in England is reliant on the women's immediate caregivers. However unreported observations (discussions with midwives and students) of routine antenatal care indicate that nutritional and weight management advice has been limited since the cessation of weighing pregnant women from the mid 1990s in England. A literature search also indicates that there have been a few weight management interventions reported.

Weight management interventions for minimising excessive weight gain during pregnancy.

There are many examples of interventions designed to manage weight when overweight and obese across a range of ages and different groups in the general, but non-pregnant, population (Luszczynska et al 2007; Counterweight Project Team 2008 for example). These include initiatives such as changing lifestyle behaviours including diet, exercise habits, and a combination of diet and exercise (Shaw et al 2006). Many initiatives including diet and/or exercise incorporate a model of behaviour change theory in the design (Cowan et al 1995; Palmeira et al 2007; Counterweight Project Team 2008). In England, weight management schemes may be funded by public and private partners and delivered free of charge or subsidised for recipients, for example, the NHS and Local Authorities (the MEND programme http:// www.mendprogramme.org/), or by commercial organisations such as Weight Watchers who have an attendance fee. Other weight management initiatives include prescribed medication such as Orlistat and Sibutramine (Neovius et al 2008), and bariatric surgery (Reedy 2009). It is also recognised that overweight/obese individuals often use low-calorie diets (Atkins and GI diets for example), accessed online information and read self-help books. Non-prescribed medication, complementary therapies and herbal remedies may also be used to aid weight loss (Amariles et al 2006).

Guidance related to obesity management in the general population to support the statutory, private and voluntary sector in England was published by NICE at the end of 2006 (NICE 2006).

At the time of writing, there have only been a few published weight management interventions related to pregnant women. This is not surprising as it is unadvisable to restrict protein and energy intake when pregnant, because of potential risks to the developing fetus and mother (Kramer and Kakuma 2003). Thus, interventions during pregnancy focus on minimising excessive weight gain(for example (Olson et al, 2004; Asbee et al 2009) to limit the risks of obesity on maternal and fetal health. It is also expected that pregnancy weight retention after the birth will be minimised, and thus the 'obesity trajectory' that often accompanies women into middle age may be inhibited (Linne et al 2003).

These pregnancy weight management studies have been outlined in *Table 12.1* to illustrate the range of interventions used, and their outcomes. None of these interventions were carried out in the UK but in other developed countries such as North America and Scandinavia. The authors are aware of studies that are underway in the UK that aim to manage weight gain in pregnant obese women, however information is not yet available (Lavender personal communication, publication forthcoming).

In the absence of evidence-based guidance for acceptable weight gain in pregnancy, the American Institute of Medicine (IOM) (1990) guidelines on weight gain in pregnancy have been used as a benchmark (see *Table 12.2*) in these studies. All interventions provided advice on healthy diet and / or exercise habits that would limit excessive weight gain during pregnancy using varying delivery models.

A review of these interventions suggests that success in weight management during pregnancy can be achieved if sufficient support is provided. Individual, personalised consultations providing counselling and education about diet and exercise suitable for pregnant women may have some success in managing weight gain, especially if the woman's progress

Table 12.1 To illustrate published studies that aim to minimise excessive weight gain in pregnancy

Author and source	Study design	Population	Intervention	Outcomes
Gray – Donald et al (2000) **Canadian Medical Association Journal**	Prospective cohort study with an intervention group and control group. Control group were monitored before the intervention group commenced.	Cree community in Canada. Obese pregnant women who did not have diabetes before pregnancy. 112 - intervention 107 - control group	-regular dietary and exercise advice based on a review of lifestyle by nutritionists in pregnancy and at 6 weeks postpartum. -during study period, healthy lifestyle information was available in written leaflets & radio broadcasts cooking demonstrations & exercise groups were available.	There were no differences in: -diet -weight gain -plasma glucose levels measured in pregnancy -maternal weight at 6 weeks postpartum between both groups.
Polley et al (2002) **International Journal of Obesity**	Randomised controlled trial	Normal and overweight pregnant women in USA. Low income women. 57 – intervention 53 – control group	- behavioural intervention of written and oral information about healthy diet and exercise at each clinic visit that was intensified when women exceeded IOM guidelines during antenatal care. - initial consultation with staff trained in nutrition and clinical psychology. - newsletters mailed bi -weekly to enhance motivation - personalised graphs of weight gain given to illustrate weight gain.	-normal weight women were significantly less likely to exceed IOM guidelines for weight gain in pregnancy at 6 week postnatal assessment (58% reduced to 33%, p <0.05) -over weight women were more likely to exceed IOM guidelines (59% compared to 33%, p<0.09)

Olson et al (2004) *American Journal of Obstetrics and Gynecology*	Prospective cohort study with an intervention and control group.	Normal and overweight pregnant women of mixed socio economic status. Mainly rural community in USA. 179 – intervention 381 - historical control	- written information about healthy diet and exercise in pregnancy at first visit - subsequent further mailed information with tips on changing behaviour and postcards to mail back with goals set - all healthcare staff were trained in providing suitable advice during routine care.	- low income overweight women were significantly less likely to exceed IOM guidelines for weight gain (52% reduced to 33%, p<0.05)
Kinnunen et al (2007) *European Journal of Clinical Nutrition*	Controlled trial (no randomisation) Six clinics – 3 x controls and 3 x intervention sites.	Under, normal, and over weight obese primigravid pregnant women in Finland. 49 – intervention 56 – control group	Individual counselling from public health nurses in up to 5 occasions during pregnancy for each of: - healthy diet - exercise.	There were no significant differences between intervention and control groups in respect of exceeding IOM guidelines for weight gain. -fibre and vegetable and fruit intake was increased in the intervention group.
Claesson et al (2008a) *British Journal of Obstetrics and Gynaecology*	Prospective cohort study with an intervention group and control group.	Obese pregnant women in Sweden. 155 – intervention 193 – control group	- individual weekly motivational talks with trained midwives where diet and exercise knowledge and habits were explored in sessions lasting around 30 minutes. - attendance at aqua natal classes (once/twice weekly) specifically designed for obese pregnant women.	-women in the intervention group had a significantly lower weight gain than those in the control group - 35.7% of women in the intervention group gained less than 7kgs compared to 20% in the control group. (p<0.003)

Wolffe et al (2008) *International Journal of Obesity*	Randomised controlled trial	Obese pregnant women in Denmark (non diabetic and non smoking) 27 – intervention 23 – control group	- 10 individual consultations lasting around an hour each with a dietician reviewing healthy diet and nutrition during pregnancy. - dietary supplements were given to all participants.	- women in the intervention group significantly limited their weight gain to 6.6kgs vs 13.3kgs in the control group (p<0.002). - serum samples indicate the deterioration in glucose metabolism was limited.
Asbee et al (2009) *Obstetrics & Gynecology*	Randomised controlled trial	Healthy women with BMI < 40.5 during pregnancy in USA 57 – intervention 43 – control group	- intensive counselling about diet and healthy lifestyle during pregnancy at the beginning of pregnancy with a dietician. - information on weight gain according to IOM guidelines given. - healthcare providers monitored progress at routine antenatal care – encouragement was provided if weight gain was within expectations. - lifestyle behaviour was reviewed and advice given accordingly if this was not within expectations.	- women in the intervention group gained significantly less weight than those in the control group (28.7 ¬+ - 12.5 lbs vs 35.6 + - 15.5 lbs, p< 0.01). -overweight and obese women were less likely to adhere to IOM guidelines (not significant) -adherence rates: Normal weight women: Intervention – 80% Control – 68.8% - overweight women: Intervention – 30% Control – 25% - obese women: Intervention – 33.3% Control – 20%

Table 12.2 Table to illustrate Institute of Medicine guidelines for weight gain in a singleton pregnancy

Body mass index	Recommended weight gain in kilogrammes	Recommended weight gain in pounds
Body mass index < 19.8	12.5 – 18	28 - 40
Body mass index 19.8 – 26	11.5 - 16	25 - 35
Body mass index 26 – 29	7 – 11.5	15 - 25
Body mass index > 29	> or = 6.8	> or = 15

Source: Institute of Medicine (1990) Nutrition during pregnancy Part I Weight gain Washington DC: National Academy Press.

is monitored throughout the pregnancy (Polley et al 2002; Olson et al 2004; Claesson et al 2008a, Wolffe et al 2008; Asbee et al 2009). Improvements to diet such as increased fibre and vitamin and mineral intake may also be attained (Kinnunen et al 2007). Interventions that are supplemented with mailed newsletters and activities that encourage participation such as goal setting, and individualised graphs that illustrate weight gain, may motivate women to continue (Polley et al 2002; Olson et al 2004). A feature of several interventions was frequent and regular contact with health care providers. This may have contributed to maintaining participating women's motivation to continue with the programme. A qualitative evaluation of the intervention with women who took part in Claesson et al's (2008a) study indicated that mental coaching and motivational discussions with healthcare providers were evaluated very positively (Claesson et al 2008b). Group social support with peers may also be helpful in maintaining motivation as women who attended the aqua natal exercise group specifically for obese pregnant women found this to be a good social experience (Claesson et al 2008b).

These studies indicate that maternity caregivers providing antenatal care, with relevant training and updating, may provide appropriate monitoring and subsequent support after the intervention has been initiated (Olson et al 2004; Claesson et al 2008a; Asbee et al 2009).

What does psychology have to offer?

Psychologists can offer advice and support to both maternity caregivers and the women themselves. Many of the feelings that can cause psychological distress (e.g. anxiety, depression, low self-esteem, negative body image etc) are more common in women in general, some of which can be explained by the social position of women in society (Dennerstein et al 1993). These types of psychological distress can be helped by the so called 'talking therapies', such as counselling. One of the most well researched and successful psychological therapy is 'cognitive behavioural therapy' (CBT) (Department of Health [DH] 2001). This is based on a cognitive model of depression that proposes that negative thoughts and beliefs can predispose to the development of depression. Cognitive behavioural therapy has been used to treat many of the underlying reasons for psychological distress, including anxiety, depression, panic attacks, and eating disorders.

Theories drawn from psychology have contributed greatly to interventions which aim to promote positive behaviour change and increase motivation. In obese populations interventions tend to be focused on weight control through diet and exercise. It is known that these behaviours are difficult to initiate and maintain even in non-obese populations, and that they require a great deal of motivation. A technique that is generally considered effective in promoting behaviour change, especially where there is a resistance to change, is motivational interviewing (MI). This is a directive, client-centred counselling style that seeks to help clients explore and resolve their ambivalence about behaviour change (Rollnick and Miller 1995). It was originally applied to people with addictive behaviours (e.g. alcohol, drugs) but it has now become a popular technique to use with people who have physical conditions (for example diet and healthy behaviour in diabetes), and healthy lifestyle programmes such as increasing fruit and vegetable intake (Resnicow et al 2001). The model which MI is based on is the 'transtheoretical model of behaviour change' (Prochaska and DiClemente 1984). The appeal of this model is that people can move up and down the five stages which reflect stages of motivational readiness (e.g. precontemplation, contemplation, preparation, action, maintenance). This allows for the fact that people do not necessarily move in a straight linear fashion when considering behaviour change, thus they could move back to contemplation, after being in a stage of preparation, before moving back again. In a community based randomised controlled trial to increase the uptake of exercise, three types of MI were compared with 523 adults: a brief one hour motivational interview or more intensive delivery of six sessions, with or without free vouchers for leisure activities (Harland et al 1999). The most effective intervention as measured at three months was the intensive MI with vouchers, although this was not maintained over the year. A note of caution, however, is that despite MI's increasing popularity with caregivers, the general quality of trials in physical health care settings remains inadequate. More research into MI applied to behaviour change is urgently required (Knight et al 2006).

The ability to predict which people who will or will not perform helpful behaviours (which are directed towards producing positive changes to lifestyle) has become a major area of research in a particular branch of psychology known as health psychology (Conner and Norman 2005).

Theories and models from health psychology have been drawn upon to underpin interventions that target those behaviours associated with obesity, such as poor diet and lack of exercise. One of the most well validated models is the theory of planned behaviour (TPB) (Ajzen and Fishbein 1970). This model sets out to address the relationship between attitudes and behaviour. The model assumes that people approach behaviour change in a rational manner, thinking through the pros and cons prior to engaging in an action. This framework also addresses the social context of behaviour change, by including norms and beliefs which can influence behaviour. However, models are only as good as the amount of behaviour they can predict and a meta-analysis of studies which had used the TBP found the addition of perceptions of control (perceived behavioural control-PBC) greatly strengthens the predictive power of the model (Armitage and Conner 2001). This is important because this allows the model to be extended to more complicated behaviours which are related to complex goals, and to those behaviours which are dependent on a sophisticated interaction with other behaviours e.g. healthy eating, uptake and maintenance of exercise programmes etc. This makes the model highly suited to the kind of complex interventions that are required to help obese pregnant women minimise weight gain during pregnancy and engage in healthy maintaining behaviours in the postnatal period.

What needs to be done?

Psychological support, and interventions that empower obese women to manage their weight gain during pregnancy, are clearly lacking in the health services of developed countries. Research is required that will enable maternity caregivers to plan and develop suitable support and care for this group of women. In particular, more understanding is required of the psychological impact of obesity during childbearing within the sociological context that the woman lives in. Some of the studies presented indicate that there is a relationship between depression and obesity (Onyike et al 2003; Roberts et al 2003; Simon et al 2006; Werrij et al 2006). Self-esteem and body image may also be affected when obese (Hill and Williams 1998). In obese pregnant women, prepregnant BMI, or depression in later pregnancy, may predict postpartum depression (LaCoursiere et al 2006; Clark et al 2009). Increasing pregnancy weight gain may trigger maternal eating behaviours that could be harmful to the developing fetus (DiPietro et al 2003). Situations that generate negative feelings may trigger maternal overeating (Nyman et al 2008). Some research indicates that being pregnant when obese may present an opportunity for some respite from the pressure to be slim (Wiles

1994, 1998; Fox and Yamaguchi 1997). It is clear from evidence published that psychological and sociological factors should be considered along with physiological issues when planning, and implementing, interventions that support obese women during pregnancy. Both qualitative and quantitative studies are needed to explore the both the degree of psychological distress, its sources, and potential barriers and facilitators to successful weight management interventions. Furthermore, maternity caregivers require the relevant skills to provide appropriate care. Multidisciplinary working is essential, especially involving those with psychology knowledge, and expertise when developing weight management interventions. Appropriate education also needs to be addressed.

A thorough health needs assessment of populations of obese pregnant women is essential to agree priorities and resources required (Cavanagh and Chadwick 2005). The interventions reported in *Table 12.1* reinforce the importance of considering the needs, characteristics and culture of the target population in the study design. For example, in Gray-Donald's et al (2000) study with indigenous Cree women in Canada, discussions with local women indicated that being 'plump' is a preferred state, and that exercise during pregnancy is not desirable. Locals also clearly remembered a period of significant starvation in their community, and so weight gain during pregnancy was considered to be very important. A lack of understanding of the beliefs of this population may have inhibited these women's uptake of the advice provided during the intervention. Polley et al's (2002) study was conducted in a deprived community where resources were limited. Participants struggled financially which impacted on accessing regular healthcare and thus contact with the study counsellors. In the area that they lived, transport for shopping was unreliable and many of the participants used coping strategies such as smoking, alcohol and drug misuse. Women in the study had limited knowledge about nutrition before participating in the study which ultimately may have affected the progress of counselling sessions provided.

Olson et al's (2004) study indicates that planning intervention materials to specifically target the needs of the population may render success more likely. Olson et al (2004) developed written materials at an appropriate reading age for their target population (fifth grade), and pretested the material in focus groups that consisted of women with similar characteristics to the study population. This ensured that information provided was appropriate, and realistic, to meet women's needs and expectations. Claesson et al (2008b) provide more insights into aspects of weight management interventions that may inhibit participation. Some Swedish women found the weekly meetings with the midwife too frequent, and aqua natal classes that were timed during normal working hours were difficult to attend.

Maternity care providers should remember that obese pregnant women may have had significant negative experiences from past encounters with health services, and other aspects of their life. It is important that these women feel confident and secure during maternity encounters. Obese women may be wary, and alert, to the care received. Communication skills used should be open and honest, but sensitive to their feelings (McCabe and Timmins 2006). Verbal and non-verbal communication should be non-threatening and non-patronising in all encounters (McCabe and Timmins 2006). Advice and information given should be practical and realistic for each individual. In particular, references made to body size and difficulties with the provision of care should reflect the possible feelings highlighted in the literature that obese and normal weight pregnant women may have about their changing body during the childbearing process. Privacy and dignity should be maintained at all times. Women may be encouraged to bring a family member or friend for support when meeting caregivers as women in Nyman et al's (2008) study found that this boosted their confidence.

Conclusion

Maternal obesity is a complex phenomenon. The evidence illustrates that psychological factors are as important as medical factors when considering the management of obesity in pregnancy. The management of an obese woman's pregnancy may have significant implications for her future mental health, as well as her physical health, and the future health of her child. The way forward for tackling this significant public health challenge involves a multidisciplinary team approach that encompasses all factors involved. It is important that more attention is directed to the psychological challenges that surround obesity and childbearing.

References

Ajzen I, Fishbein M (1970). The prediction of behaviour from attitudinal and normative beliefs. *Journal of Personality and Social Psychology*. **6**: 466-87

Amador N, Judrez JM, Guizar JM et al (2008) Quality of life in obese pregnant women: a longitudinal study. *American Journal of Obstetrics & Gynecology*. **198**(2):203.e1-203. e5.

Amariles P., Gonzalez LI, Giraldo NA (2006) Prevalence of self-treatment with complementary products and therapies for weight loss: a randomized cross-sectional study in overweight and obese patients in Columbia. *Current Therapeutic Research*. **67**(1):66-78.

Armitage C, Conner M (2001) Efficacy of the Theory of Planned Behaviour: A meta-analytic review. *British Journal of Social Psychology.* **40**: 471–99

Asbee SM, Jenkins TR, Butler JR et al (2009) Preventing excessive weight gain during pregnancy through dietary and lifestyle counselling. *Obestetrics & Gynecology* **113**(2) Part 1, 305-11

Cavanagh S, Chadwick K (2005) *Health needs assessment: A practical guide Health Development Agency*: **London.**

Claesson I-M, Sydsjo G, Cedergren M et al (2008a) Weight gain restriction for obese pregnant women: a case-control intervention study *BJOG* **115**:44-50

Claesson I-M, Josefsson A, Cedergren M et al (2008b) Consumer satisfaction with a weight-gain intervention programme for obese pregnant women. *Midwifery.* **24**(2):163-7

Clark MP, Ogden J (1999) The impact of pregnancy on eating behaviour and aspects of weight concern. *International Journal of Obesity.* **23`**;18-24

Clark A, Skouteris H, Wertheim EH et al (2009) The relationship between depression and body dissatisfaction across pregnancy and the postpartum A prospective study. *Journal of Health Psychology.* **14**(1):27-35.

Conner M, Norman P (2005) Predicting health behaviour. second edition. Open University Press: Berkshire, England.

Copper RL, DuBard MB, Goldenberg RL et al (1995) The relationship of maternal attitude toward weight gain to weight gain during pregnancy and low birth weight. *Obstetrics & Gynecology.* **85**(4):590-5.

Counterweight Project Team (2008) Evaluation of the Counterweight programme for obesity management in primary care: a starting point for continuous improvement. *British Journal of General Practice.* **58**,548-54.

Cowan R, Britton PJ, Logue E et al (1995) The relationship among the transtheoretical model of behavioral change, psychological distress, and diet attitudes in obesity: Implications for primary care intervention *Journal of Clinical Psychology in Medical Settings.* **2**(3):249-67.

Dennerstein L, Astbury J, Morse C (1993) P*sychosocial and mental health aspects of women's health. Geneva, Switzerland, World Health Organization*, 4, 97 p. (WHO/FHE/MNH/93.1).

Department of Health (2001) *Treatment Choice in Psychological Therapies and Counselling. Evidence Based Clinical Practice Guidelines.* DH:London.

Di Pietro JA, Millett S, Costigan KA et al (2003) Psychosocial influences on weight gain attitudes and behaviors during pregnancy. *Journal of the American Dietetic Association.* **103**(10):1314-19.

Fox P Yamaguchi C (1997) Body image change in pregnancy: A comparison of normal weight and overweight primigravidas *Birth.* **24**(1):35-40.

Friedman KE, Reichmann SK, Costanzo PR et al (2005) Weight stigmatization and ideological beliefs: Relation to psychological functioning in obese adults. *Obesity Research*. **13**(5):907-16.

Furber C, Garrod DG, Maloney E et al (2007) *Pregnant women's experiences of psychological distress: An exploratory study*. Report to Queen's Nursing Institute: University of Manchester: Manchester.

Gray-Donald K, Robinson E, Collier A et al (2000) Intervening to reduce weight gain in pregnancy and gestational diabetes mellitus in Cree communities: an evaluation. *Canadian Medical Association Journal* **163**(10):1247-73

Greenberg, B.S, Eastin M., Hofschire L.et al (2003) Portrayals of overweight and obese individual on commercial television *American Journal of Public Health* **93** (8): 1342-48.

Harland J, White M, Drinkwater C et al (1999). The Newcastle exercise project: a randomised controlled trial of methods to promote physical activity in primary care. *British Medical Journal* **319**: 828-32.

Hill AJ and Williams J (1998) Psychological health in a non-clinical sample of obese women. *International Journal of Obesity*. **22**: 578-83.

Institute of Medicine (1990) *Nutrition during pregnancy Part 1 Weight gain* Washington DC: National Academy Press.

Johnson S, Burrows A, Williamson I. (2004) 'Does my bump look good in this?' The meaning of bodily changes for first-time mothers-to-be. *Journal of Health Psychology* **9**(3): 361-74.

Kinnunen TI, Pasanen M, Aittasalo M et al (2007) Preventing excessive weight gain during pregnancy – a controlled trial in primary health care *European Journal of Clinical Nutrition* **61**, 884-91.

Knight KM, Mcgowan L, Dickens C et al (2006) A systematic review of motivational interviewing in physical health care settings. *British Journal of Health Psychology* **11**(2):319-32.

Kramer MS, Kakuma R. Energy and protein intake in pregnancy. Cochrane Database of Systematic Reviews 2003, Issue 4. Art. No.: CD000032. DOI: 10.1002/14651858. CD000032.

LaCoursiere DY, Baksh L, Bloeman L et al (2006) Maternal body mass index and self - reported postpartum depressive symptoms. *Maternal and Child Health Journal*. **10**(4):385-90

Linne Y, Dye L, Barkeling B. et al (2003) Weight development over time in parous women – The SPAWN study – 15 years follow-up *International Journal of Obesity* **27**,1516-22.

Luszczynska A, Sobczyk A, Abraham C (2007) Planning to lose weight: Randomized controlled trial of an implementation intention prompt to enhance weight reduction among overweight and obese women. *Health Psychology*. **26**(4):507-12.

McCabe C, Timmins F (2006) *Communications skills for nursing practice*. Palgrave

Macmillan: New York.

Merrill E Grassley J (2008) Women's stories of their experiences as overweight patients. *Journal of Advanced Nursing.* **64**(2):139-46.

Miller W R, Rollnick S (1991). *Motivational interviewing: Preparing people to change addictive behaviour.* Guildford Press: New York.

Neovius M, Johansson K, Rossner S (2008) Head-to-head studies evaluating efficacy of pharmaco-therapy for obesity: a systematic review and meta-analysis. *Obesity Reviews.* :420-27.

NICE (2006) *Obesity: the prevention, identification, assessment and management of overweight and obesity in adults and children.* NICE:London.

NICE (2007) *Antenatal and Postnatal Mental Health* NICE: London.

NICE (2008) *Antenatal care Routine care for the healthy pregnant woman* RCOG: London.

Nyman VMK, Prebensen AK, Flensner GEM (2008) Obese women's experiences of encounters with midwives and physicians during pregnancy and childbirth. *Midwifery.* Doi:101016/j.midw.2008.10.008.

Olsen CM, Strawderman MS, Reed RG (2004) Efficacy of an intervention to prevent excessive gestational weight gain *American Journal of Obstetrics and Gynecology* **191** 530-6.

Onyike CU, Crum RM, Lee HB et al (2003) Is obesity associated with major depression? Results from the Third National Health and Nutrition Examination Survey. *American Journal of Epidemiology.* **158**(12):1139-42.

Palmeira A L, Teixeira PJ, Branco TL et al (2007) Predicting short-term weight loss using four leading health behaviour change theories *International Journal of Behavioural Nutrition and Physical Activity.* **4**(14):doi:10.1186/1479-5868-4-14.

Polley BA Wing RR Sims CJ (2002) Randomized controlled trial to prevent excessive weight gain in pregnant women *International Journal of Obesity* **26**: 1494-1502

Prochaska J DiClemente C (1984). The transtheoretical approach: Crossing traditional boundaries of therapy. Krieger:Malabar, FL.

Puhl R and Brownell KD (2001) Bias, stigma, and discrimination. *Obesity Research.* **9**(12): 788-805.

Puhl R and Brownell KD (2003) Psychosocial origins of obesity stigma: toward changing a powerful and pervasive bias. *Obesity Reviews.* **4**:213-27.

Puhl R, Moss-Racusin CA, Schwartz MB et al (2008) Weight stigmatization and bias reduction: perspectives of overweight and obese adults. *Health Education Research.* **23**(2):347-58.

Reedy S (2009) An evidence-based review of obesity and bariatric surgery. *Journal of Nurse-Practitioners.* **5**(1):22-9.

Resnicow K, Jackson A, Want T et al (2001). A motivational interviewing intervention to increase fruit and vegetable intake through black churches: Results of the eat for life trial. *American Journal of Public Health* **91:** 1686–93.

Ritchie J and Spencer E (1994) *Qualitative data analysis for applied policy research*. In Bryman A Burgess RG (eds.) Analyzing Qualitative Data. Routledge: London.

Roberts RE, Deleger S, Strawbridge WJ et al (2003) Prospective association between obesity and depression: evidence from the Alamada County Study. *International Journal of Obesity*. **27**:514-21.

Rollnick S and Miller W R (1995). What is motivational interviewing? *Behavioural and Cognitive Psychotherapy*. **23**(4): 325–34.

Shaw K, Gennat H, O'Rourke P et al Exercise for overweight or obesity. *Cochrane Database of Systematic Reviews 2006,* Issue 4. Art. No.: CD003817. DOI: 10.1002/14651858.CD003817.pub3.

Simon GE, Von Korff M, Saunders K et al (2006) Association between obesity and psychotic disorders in the US adult population. *Archives of General Psychiatry*. **63**:824-30.

Skouteris H, Carr R, Wertheim EH et al (2005) A prospective study of factors that lead to body dissatisfaction during pregnancy. *Body Image*. **2**: 347-61.

Stevens-Simon C, Nakashima II, Andrews D (1993) Weight gain attitudes among pregnant adolescents. *Journal of Adolescent Health* **14**:369-72.

Strang VR and Sullivan PL (1985) Body image attitudes during pregnancy and the postpartum period. *Journal of Obstetric Gynecologic and Neonatal Nursing*. July/ August 332-37.

Thomas S, Hyde J, Karunaratne A et al (2008) Being 'fat' in today's world: a qualitative study of the lived experiences of people with obesity in Australia. *Health Expectations*. **11**(4):321-30.

Warriner S (2000) Women's views of being weighed during pregnancy. *British Journal of Midwifery* **8**(10):620-23.

Werrij Q, Mulkens S, Hospers HJ et al (2006) Overweight and obesity: The significance of a depressed mood. *Patient Education and Counselling*. **62**,126-31.

Wiles, R. (1994) *'I'm not fat, I'm pregnant': The impact of pregnancy on fat women's body image In*: Wilkinson, S., Kitzinger, C. (Eds.) (1994) Women and Health Feminist Perspectives. Taylor & Francis: Bristol. Chapter 3.

Wiles, R. (1998) The views of women of above average weight about appropriate weight gain in pregnancy. *Midwifery*. **14**:254-60.

Wolff S, Legarth J, Vangaard K et al (2008) A randomized controlled trial of the effects of dietary counselling on gestational weight gain and glucose metabolism in obese pregnant women. *International Journal of Obesity*. **32**:495-501.

Chapter 13

Obesity: Lessons Learned from the Confidential Enquiries Into Maternal Deaths Report 2003 -2005

Asma Khalil and Pat O'Brien

The Confidential Enquiries into Maternal and Child Health (CEMACH), which at time of publication was to be renamed the Centre for Maternal and Child Enquiries (CMACE), is the longest running audit into national maternal mortality in the world. Its triennial reports audit all maternal deaths in the UK during the preceding three years, search for causes and associations, and for lessons to be learned. The most recent report covered the period from 2003 to 2005 (Lewis 2007). The overall maternal mortality rate was 13.95 per 100,000 maternities - a total of 295 women out of more than 2 million maternities; the leading causes of direct and indirect deaths are shown in *Table 13.1*. The association between obesity and many of the leading causes of maternal death, such as cardiac disease, thromboembolic disease, pre eclampsia (PE), sepsis and haemorrhage, has long been recognised (Kanagalingam et al 2005, Lashen et al 2004, Weiss et al 2004, Usha et al 2005, Myles 2002). Obesity also increases the risk of gestational diabetes, complicates anaesthesia (both regional and general, particularly in pregnant women) and increases the likelihood of Caesarean section (CS) (Kanagalingam et al 2005, Lashen et al 2004, Weiss et al 2004, Usha et al 2005, Myles 2002). As well as the increased risk to the mother, the babies of obese women are also at increased risk of a number of complications including congenital fetal anomaly, prematurity, stillbirth and neonatal death (Ray et al 2005, Watkins et al 2003, Cedegren and Kallen 2003, Cedegren and Kallen 2005, Stephensson et al 2001, Kristensen 2005). It is not surprising, therefore, that obesity is viewed as a significant and growing contributor to maternal mortality both in the UK and world-wide.

Table 13.1 Rates per 100 000 maternities of maternal deaths reported to CEMACH by cause; United Kingdom: 2003-2005			
Rates per 100 000 maternities	Direct		Indirect
1	Thromboembolism	1.94	Cardiac	2.27
2	Pre eclampsia/eclampsia	0.85	Psychiatric Indirect	0.85
3	Genital tract sepsis*	0.85		
4	Amniotic fluid embolus	0.80		
5	Haemorrhage	0.66		
Total	All Direct	6.24	All Indirect 7.71	
	*includes early pregnancy deaths due to sepsis			

Table 13.2 Classification of Body Mass Index (BMI)		
BMI (kg/m²)	BMI classification (Information Centre Health and Social Care 2006)	NICE classification (2006)
Under 18.5	Underweight	
18.5 – 24.9	Normal	Healthy weight
25.0 – 29.9	Overweight	Overweight
30.0 – 34.9	Obese	Obesity I
35.0 – 39.9		Obesity II
40.0 or over	Morbidly obese	Obesity III

CEMACH Report 2003 to 2005

Various classifications of BMI are available (*Table 13.2*). For the purposes of the most recent CEMACH report (Lewis 2007), obesity in pregnancy was defined as a BMI of 30 or greater at booking. Documentation of BMI was quite good in the second half of pregnancy but less so in the first half; there was a failure to record BMI in only 18 of the women who died after 22 weeks' gestation compared with 46 of the women who died before 22 weeks. More than half (52%) of all the women who died from either direct or indirect causes, and for whom BMI was known, were either overweight or obese. This proportion was similar for direct (55%) and indirect (49%) deaths. In fact, around one in six of all women who died were either morbidly or super-morbidly obese: 15% of those who died and whose BMI was known had a BMI greater than 35, half of whom had a BMI greater than 40. A further 36% of women had BMIs between 25 and 34 (12% between 30 and 34, and 24% between 25 and 29).

Limitations of the CEMACH Report

All of the data presented above suggest that obesity may play a significant role in maternal mortality in the United Kingdom, and certainly previous studies have established links between obesity and many of the major causes of maternal mortality. However, a significant limitation of the CEMACH reports, and one which is acknowledged within the reports themselves, is the lack of good population data for comparison. In particular, there are no reliable up to date national data describing the BMI or rates of obesity in pregnant women in the UK. The best data available on obesity in the general population (not specifically pregnant) in the UK are collected for the Health Surveys for England, the longest data series on this topic (Information Centre for Health and Clinical Excellence 2006). These data suggest a steady rise in obesity rates in the general population between 1993 and 2005; during this time, the proportion of women with a BMI between 30.1 and 40.0 rose from 15.0% to 19.0%, and women with a BMI over 40 rose from 1.4% to 2.9%. Similarly, Kanagalingam et al's (2005) study of pregnant women in Glasgow, Scotland, described a significant increase in obesity rates among pregnant women over more than a decade (assessed in 1990 and 2002/2004). Several cross sectional studies have described obesity rates ranging between 11% and 20% of the pregnant population in the UK (Information Centre for Health and Clinical Excellence 2006, Sebire et al 2001, Shah et al 2006). Because of the limited information on obesity rates in the general pregnant population, it is not possible to calculate BMI-specific maternal mortality rates. It is therefore impossible to draw accurate conclusions about the influence of obesity on the relative risk of maternal death from all causes or associated with individual complications.

Nevertheless, it does seem clear that obesity rates in the UK general female and pregnant populations have risen steadily over the past 10 to 15 years, and it is known from other studies that obesity is associated with an increased risk of many of the leading causes of maternal death. It is postulated, therefore, that the lack of a fall in maternal mortality rates in the UK over the past decade may be explained by the fact that the pregnant population is more obese, older and has an increasing number of medical complications. The Health Surveys for England (Information Centre for Health and Clinical Excellence 2006) confirmed something not entirely unexpected: in women, BMI increases with age, a trend which is apparent through the childbearing years. For example, the proportion of women with a BMI between 30.1 - 40.0 increases from 11.1% in the age group 16-24 years, to 15.1% in the age group 25-34 years, to 18.6% in the age group 35-44 years.

The lack of good national data on obesity levels in the general pregnant population has led CEMACH to institute a national audit of care provided to women with a BMI of 35 and over (see overleaf).

Thromboembolic disease

Of the 31 women who died with thromboembolic disease and had a known BMI, 14 were obese.

> *"A morbidly obese woman required a wheelchair because she weighed almost 200 kg at the end of her pregnancy. Correctly she was assessed antenatally by the anaesthetist and excellent care was provided when fetal distress developed in labour and a Caesarean section was required. She had thromboprophylaxis (Tinzaparin 5000 units daily) and was discharged within a week of delivery. Shortly afterwards she complained of breathlessness but this was attributed to her obesity. She died a few days later."*

The CEMACH Report concludes that in this case "although the general care provided for this woman was excellent, she presented a very difficult problem... the prophylactic dose of Tinzaparin was appropriate for normal body weight but the RCOG guideline recommends 4500 units twelve hourly for a woman with a body weight over 90 kg".

The Report noted substandard care in only one case of cerebral vein thrombosis, compared with two thirds (22 of 33) of cases of pulmonary embolism. The main areas of substandard care were:

- Inadequate risk assessment in early pregnancy.
- A failure to recognise or act on risk factors.
- A failure to appreciate the significance of signs and symptoms in women who had known risk factors.
- A failure to initiate treatment promptly.
- A failure to use adequate doses of thromboprophylactic drugs.

The Report noted that in spite of increasing risk factors (increasing rates of obesity, more and further air travel, a rise in the age of women becoming pregnant and a rise in CS rates), the number of maternal deaths from thromboembolism had shown no significant change for 20 years. The Report suggests that this is due to increasing vigilance and awareness among obstetricians and midwives, and the use of guidelines for thromboprophylaxis in pregnancy, particularly peripartum. In fact there has been a *fall* in deaths from pulmonary embolism following CS during that time. However, the Report recommends that the same level of awareness and vigilance is also required in early pregnancy and following vaginal delivery. It notes, for example, that of the 10 women who died in the first trimester, seven had identifiable risk factors, and four were obese or morbidly obese. Therefore, the Report highlights the need for prepregnancy counselling to be made accessible to obese women. It also cautions against "inappropriate classification" of obese women as 'low risk' in pregnancy and recommends that: "all women should undergo an assessment of risk factors in early pregnancy or before pregnancy. This assessment should be repeated if the woman is admitted to hospital or develops other intercurrent problems".

Sepsis

This CEMACH Report identifies a long list of factors associated with an increased risk of sepsis, which includes obesity, diabetes, impaired immunity, anaemia and CS. One case noted:

"A woman collapsed and died due to pulmonary embolism. She had several risk factors for this including obesity, laparotomy for primary PPH, suboptimal thromboprophylaxis and vaginal sepsis due to inadvertent retention of a tampon inserted during repair of a vaginal tear. Vaginal examination was extremely difficult because of her high BMI which was over 35. She had offensive lochia but the tampon remained undiscovered despite several vaginal examinations until it was extruded a month later."

This case highlights how obesity can increase the risk of sepsis and compound other complications.

Anaesthesia

Around half (150) of all women who died in this triennium had had an anaesthetic, but the assessors considered that only six had died from problems directly associated with anaesthesia. Of these six women who died directly due to anaesthetic complications, four were obese, two of whom were morbidly obese.

"An obese asthmatic woman died as a result of failed re-intubation during the recovery phase after anaesthesia for laparoscopic surgery for an ectopic pregnancy. She developed acute respiratory distress due to severe bronchospasm on extubation. A senior anaesthetist was called but by then she had suffered an irreversible cardiac arrest."

"A morbidly obese asthmatic woman had an elective CS for which a consultant anaesthetist administered spinal anaesthesia. She became agitated and short of breath after surgery but she was sent to the postnatal ward a few hours later. She received oxygen but remained agitated and short of breath. She was reviewed by an anaesthetist but had a fatal cardiac arrest a few hours later. There were additional problems with the ready availability of resuscitation equipment on the postnatal ward."

This Report highlights the difficulty in administering either regional or general anaesthesia to obese pregnant women. It also expressed concern that anaesthetic trainees are now less experienced than before in laryngoscopy, intubation and other advanced airway techniques, particularly in pregnant women. The Report derives the following learning points with regard to anaesthesia in obese pregnant women:

● All obstetric units should have a protocol for the management of obese pregnant women; this protocol should include a section on anaesthesia which should deal with pre-assessment procedures, special equipment such as large sphygmomanometer cuffs, hoists, beds and operating tables, and long regional block needles.

● Morbidly obese women should be referred to an anaesthetist during the pregnancy for an anaesthetic assessment.

● Difficulties with airway management and intubation should be anticipated, so these women should be managed by a consultant anaesthetist.

● Extra manpower is often required to position the woman correctly for induction of general anaesthesia.

● In morbidly obese women, sphygmomanometry is often inaccurate, so consideration should be given to using direct arterial pressure measurements during surgical procedures.

● With regard to thromboprophylactic low molecular weight heparin, a dose appropriate to the woman's weight should be used and duration of therapy should take into account the degree and duration of immobility. Thromboembolic stockings of appropriate size should be made available.

Acquired heart disease

Sixteen women died from myocardial infarction and/or ischaemic heart disease, representing a fourfold increase compared to the previous triennium (Lewis 2007). The assessors felt that this was probably associated with increasing maternal age, obesity and smoking in pregnancy. Six of the 16 were morbidly obese with a BMI of 35 or more; four of these six had a BMI over 40. A similar proportion of women who died from hypertensive heart disease or sudden adult death syndrome (SADS) were obese. The Report highlighted the well-recognised links between abdominal obesity, the metabolic syndrome and increased cardiovascular risk.

"A multiparous, obese woman was prescribed clomiphene for infertility. Her booking BP was high and thereafter her hypertension was

suboptimally controlled. She also developed gestational diabetes. Her GP prescribed salbutamol for "wheezing". An echocardiogram was suboptimal. Postnatally, there was inadequate monitoring of her BP and the midwives did not appreciate the significance of a "rattly" chest and chest pain. She died of hypertensive heart failure five days after delivery. Autopsy revealed a grossly enlarged heart with left and right ventricular hypertrophy, and evidence of longstanding back pressure on the lungs and congestive cardiac failure."

This case highlights the importance of prepregnancy counselling about the risks of obesity in pregnancy, as well as the risk of hypertensive heart disease and the importance of careful investigation of cardiac or respiratory symptoms in obese women during pregnancy.

The logistical problems associated with obesity

Apart from the clear association with many complications of pregnancy for the woman and her baby as described above, this CEMACH Report also highlighted many logistical problems associated with obesity in pregnancy. Obesity carries an increased risk of congenital fetal anomalies; this is compounded by the fact that prenatal diagnosis, both ultrasound scan and invasive testing, is often more difficult. Obesity increases the risk of delay in diagnosis, for example of ectopic pregnancy or deep vein thrombosis. Pre-existing dyspnoea and/or orthopnoea may mask cardiac or respiratory symptoms. The Report cites one case in which a woman's resuscitation was delayed because the ambulance services were unable to remove her from her home. In one woman, the diagnosis of pre eclampsia was made late because of a lack of suitably sized sphygmomanometer cuffs. Several CS had to be performed on two beds pushed together because the operating table was unable to bear the weight of the woman; clearly this was suboptimal.

The Report describes the cases of two morbidly obese women who died in the first trimester. One avoided doctors and midwives completely; the Report states that this highlighted the fact that obese women may be embarrassed about their condition and fearful of stigmatisation, and doctors and midwives must be sensitive to these feelings. The second woman, who also had a thrombophilia, booked early but died before seeing the haematologist to whom she had been referred. This led the CEMACH assessors to recommend that such high risk obese women should be treated as emergencies. Ideally, they should be counselled and, where appropriate, management commenced prior to pregnancy.

Recommendations

Apart from many topic-based recommendations, some of which are mentioned above, the Report also makes some overarching recommendations with regard to obesity in pregnancy:

1. Prepregnancy counselling, both targeted and opportunistic, should be made available to obese women of childbearing age. This applies particularly to women undergoing assisted reproduction or fertility investigations. Such prepregnancy counselling about the risks of obesity in pregnancy would probably lead to some women avoiding pregnancy. Others would be encouraged to lose weight and improve their general health prior to conceiving. All counselled women would be fully aware of the risks, would be more likely to seek early referral once pregnancy is confirmed, would start prophylactic measures (where appropriate) early and would be aware of the warning symptoms for which they should be vigilant.

2. The Report highlights the need for a national guideline specific to the management of obesity in pregnancy. Although there is a National Institute for Health and Clinical Excellent (NICE) (2006) guideline on the management of obesity in children and adults, there is no guideline specific to obese pregnant women.

3. All obese women who fall pregnant should be referred for early multi-disciplinary planning regarding mode of delivery, anaesthesia and thromboprophylaxis.

Future Research for CEMACH

This Report recognises the increasing prevalence of obesity in the UK and the fact that obesity increases the risk of maternal death. More than half of all women who died, for whom information about BMI was available, were either overweight or obese, and more than 15% were morbidly or super-morbidly obese. In response to this, CEMACH has undertaken a national Obesity in Pregnancy Project which is planned to run from 2008 until 2010. This project consists of three phases:

Phase 1: A national survey investigating how well maternity units are equipped to care for women with obesity.

Phase 2: The development of national standards of care based on evidence and consensus expert opinion.

Phase 3: A national audit of care provided to women with BMI over 35.

The guideline for managing obesity in pregnancy has recently been published (Phase 2) (Modder and Fitzsimons 2010). This initiative taken by CEMACH should dovetail well with the work being done by the United Kingdom Obstetric Surveillance System (UKOSS) since 2007 investigating:
a) the prevalence of extreme obesity in pregnancy in the UK
b) the risk of adverse outcomes attributable to extreme obesity in pregnancy
c) any adverse outcomes relating to inadequate weight capacity equipment.

Conclusion

It seems clear from CEMACH Reports, particularly the most recent (2005 to 2008), that obesity is a major contributing factor to several complications leading to maternal death. In addition, obesity poses a number of logistical problems which also increase the risk. However, because of the lack of good quality data on the prevalence of obesity in the general pregnant population, CEMACH has been unable to accurately quantify these relative risks. Future research by both CEMACH and UKOSS will help to address these issues. In the meantime, many of the recommendations of the 2003-2005 CEMACH Report, both general and specific, are eminently sensible and should be addressed by all Maternity Units in the UK.

References

Cedegran MI, Kallen BA (2003) Maternal obesity and infant heart defects. *Obes Res* **11**:1065-71.

Cedegran MI, Kallen BA (2005) Maternal obesity and the risk of orofacial clefts in the offspring. *Cleft Palate Craniofac J*;42:367-71.

Information Centre for Health and Social Care (2006) *Statistics on obesity, physical activity and diet: England, 2006*. Leeds: Information Centre.

Kanagalingam MG, Forouhi NG, Greer IA et al (2005) Changes in booking body mass index over a decade: retrospective analysis from a Glasgow Maternity Hospital. *BJOG* **112**:1431-3.

Kristensen J, Vestergaard M, Wisborg K, et al (2005) Pre-pregnancy weight and the risk of stillbirth and neonatal death. *BJOG* **112**:403-8.

Lashen H, Fear K, Sturdee DW (2005) Obesity is associated with increased risk of first trimester and recurrent miscarriage: matched case control study. *Hum Reprod* **19**:1644-6.

Lewis, G (ed) 2007. *The Confidential Enquiry into Maternal and Child Health (CEMACH). Saving Mothers' Lives: reviewing maternal deaths to make motherhood safer 2003*

2005. The Seventh Report on Confidential Enquiries into Maternal Deaths in the United Kingdom. London: CEMACH.

Modder J, Fitzsimons KJ (2010) *CMACE/RCOG Joint Guideline: Management of Women with Obesity in Pregnancy*. London: CMACE & RCOG.

Myles TD, Gooch J, Santolaya J (2005) Obesity is an independent risk factor for infectious morbidity in patients who undergo caesarean delivery. *Obstet Gynecol* **100**;959-64.

National Institute for Health and Clinical Excellence (2006). *Obesity: the prevention, identification, assessment and management of overweight and obesity in adults and children*. National Institute for Health and Clinical Excellence (NICE), 2006. http://www.nice.org.uk/guidance/CG43

Ray JG, Wyatt PR, Vermuelen MJ et al (2005) Greater maternal weight and the ongoing risk of neural tube defects after folic acid flour fortification. *Obstet Gynecol* **105**:261-5.

Sebire NJ, Jolly M, Harris JP et al (2001) Maternal obesity and pregnancy outcome: a study of 287,213 pregnancies in London. *Int J Obes Relat Metab Disord* **25**:1175-82.

Shah A, Sands J, Kenny L (2006) Maternal obesity and the risk of stillbirth and neonatal death. *J Obstet Gynaecol* **26** I (Suppl 1)S19. 2005.

Stephansson O, Dickman PW, Johansson A et al (2001) Maternal weight, pregnancy weight gain, and the risk of antepartum stillbirth. *Am J Obstet Gynecol* **184**:463-9.

Usha KTS, Hemmadi J, Bethel J et al (2005) Outcome of pregnancy in women with an increased body mass index. *BJOG* **112**:768-72.

Watkins ML, Rasmussen SA, Honein MA et al (2003) Maternal obesity and risk for birth defects. *Paediatrics* **111**:1152-8.

Weiss JL, Malone FD, Emig D et al (2004) Obesity, obstetric complications and cesarean delivery rate - a population based screening study. *Am J Obstet Gynecol* **190**:1091-7.

Index